GROW HAIR

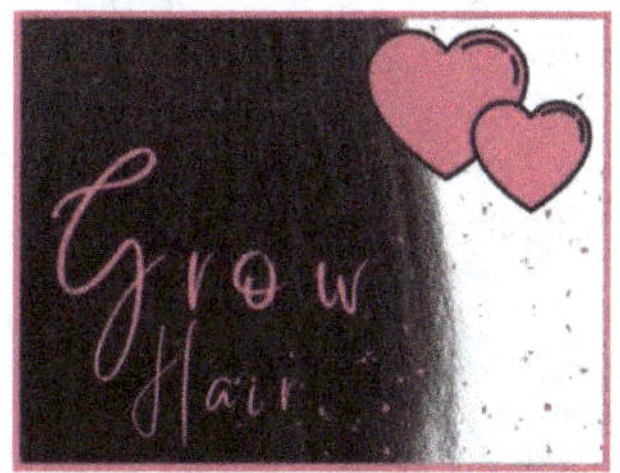

A Complete Guide to Retaining, Maintaining and Growing African Hair

My dear lovely lady, there is no one else who is just like you. Your uniqueness makes you beautiful. Believe it! Embrace your essence...

Michelle Layla Ismael

Disclaimer:
This book is not intended as a substitute for the medical advice of physicians. You should consult a physician in matters relating to the health of your hair or scalp and particularly with respect to any symptoms that may require diagnosis or medical attention. The author and publisher advise readers to take full responsibility for their hair and know their limits. Before practicing the skills described in this book, be sure that your products and equipment is well maintained and of high quality. Do not take risks beyond your level of experience, aptitude, training, and comfort level.

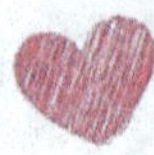  

Dedication

To my daughter Gabby, who taught me to love our crown of glory, which is our natural African textured hair.

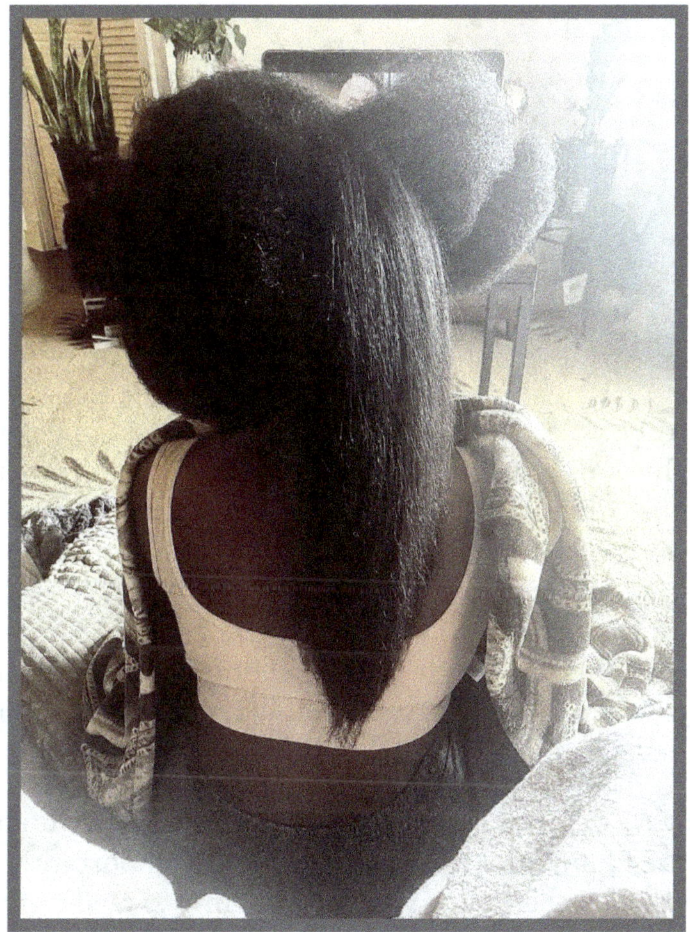

Gabby's hair blow dried straight (Full blow dry)

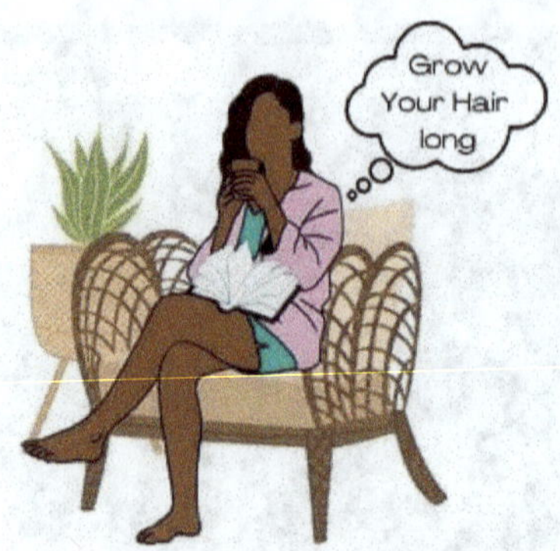

It is truly a pleasure that you have an interest in beginning a healthy hair routine and growing your hair to very long lengths. First, I would like to congratulate you for not believing that your hair cannot grow and seeking information on how to grow it longer than you ever have before. The most difficult part about growing long hair is waiting for it to get long. However, like every goal in life, it is about your perception. If you take the time to treat your hair with care now, you will not regret or wish that you had years from now.

This is a very detailed guide that will help you better understand the basics of hair, how to grow it, and most importantly how to take care of it. Please allow yourself the time to read it if your ultimate goal is to have long and healthy hair.

Now I'll tell you a little bit about my hair journey...

I started relaxing my hair at about age 12. At first my hair was beautiful, shiny and thick, but with each relaxer, it appeared thinner. After 15 years of relaxing my hair, and never having a haircut, my hair stayed the same length and I saw *zero* growth. In fact, by the time I was 20, my hair was thin, see-through, breaking and not growing beyond my shoulders. I had very thin edges and no hair in the back of my head.

After I had my son in 2010, I began educating myself on how to grow my relaxed hair long. I tried every technique, but my hair continued to break. One evening, my mother saw me looking at several YouTube videos of relaxed women styling their waist length hair. She looked at me with concern and said, *"You need to stop giving yourself hope, because long hair is not in your DNA"*. She was right, my type of hair was not typical for this type of growth, but I was determined to prove that theory wrong.

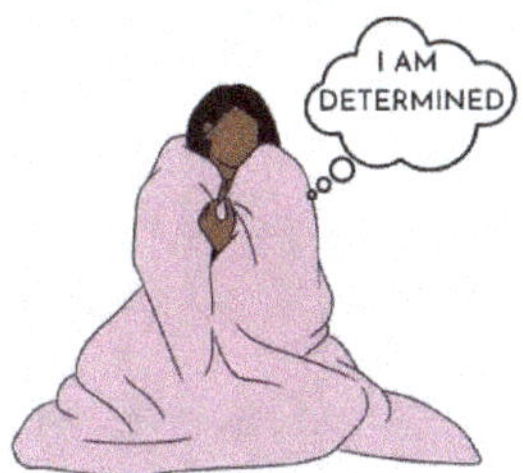

At that very moment, I made up my mind to stop relaxing and wear my hair natural. My natural hair wasn't the *soft or good* hair. It was the kinkiest of all kinky hair. There was not a lot of information about how to grow my kind of hair long. I thought *going natural* and wearing braids was all there was to growing my hair long and I continued with my old habits of not really taking proper care of my hair. In the back of my mind, I kept hoping, but not really believing, that my hair would ever grow long.

One day as I sat looking at my daughter's hair, which looked just like mine, I came to the realization that God gave us African textured hair and I did not love, appreciate, or take proper care of this gift. In fact, I had tried everything to change the way my hair looked. It was then that I began praying for long hair. I prayed that with the proper care, God will give me the grace to allow me and my hair to glorify him.

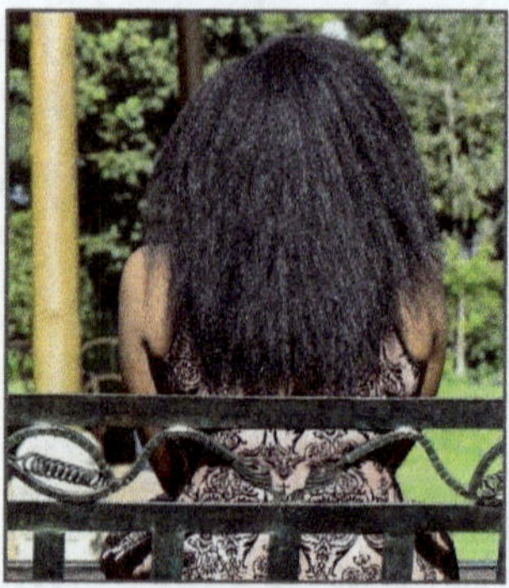

My hair is now longer than it has ever been and with those practices, I was also able to grow my daughter's hair to her waist. This is why I know that if I can do it, you can too.

Michelle

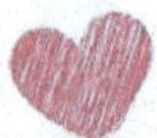  

And God made everything beautiful in its own time...

ECCLESIASTES 3:11

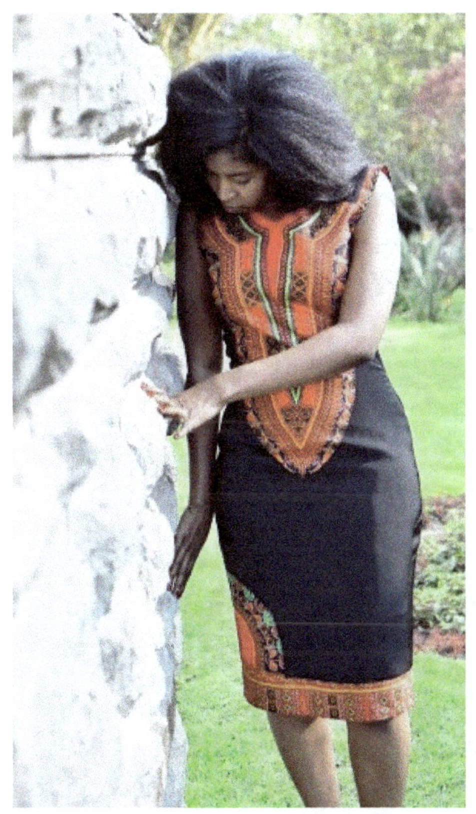

CHAPTER 1

7 Things You Thought Were True About Your Hair (But Are False)

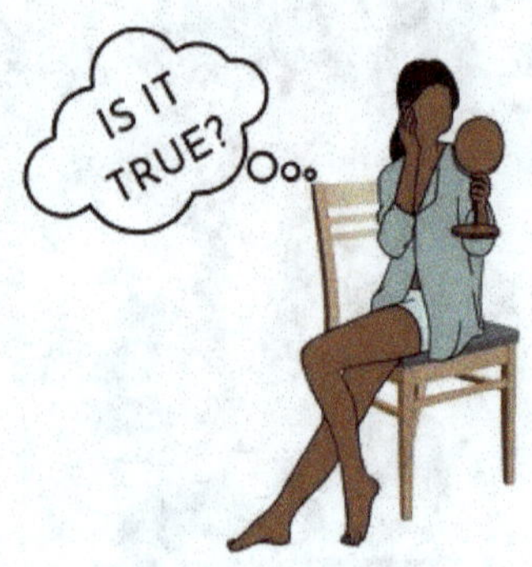

To start, you will often hear people say…

1) African textured hair is ugly – False.

Who taught you that your hair is ugly? Who taught you that your hair is an embarrassment and it needed to be covered up or straight to be beautiful? God made all things beautiful. Does that mean that he made a mistake with your hair? Once you discover how beautiful and versatile your hair is, you will fall in love with it to the point where you will not want to stop touching it. Know that your hair is a gift from God and with this appreciation you will see your crown of glory that he has intended for you to have.

If you wear your hair confidently, others will also appreciate your hair. A confident woman is a beautiful woman. African textured hair is beautiful hair. Your hair is the only hair type that can be an afro today, curly tomorrow, and straight the next day.

2) African textured hair cannot grow long, only women with "good" hair can grow long hair - False.

You CAN grow your hair long. When you learn how to practice proper hair care, you can keep the hair that is already growing from your scalp. Good hair is healthy hair and healthy "hard" hair is good hair.

3) Long hair is due to family background - False.

Family background can determine how fast and how long your hair can grow, but how you *care* for your hair determines how much of it you will *keep* and therefore how *long* it can be.

4) Natural African textured hair is the strongest hair - False.

Remove a strand of your hair and recognize the many bends and twists that it has. These bends and twists are the parts that are weaker, which makes African textured hair the weakest of all other racial groups. This is why to grow long hair, gentle care should be practiced to avoid damage.

5) There are products that can repair damaged hair - False.

Damaged hair is like damaged nails which cannot be repaired, only trimmed off to prevent future splitting and breakage.

6) Natural hair is difficult to work with and maintain - False.

Once you have learned the proper techniques, natural hair is much easier to maintain than chemically treated hair that requires extreme maintenance for the average woman to grow long hair.

7) Natural Hair means that you are too poor to fix it – False.

Women all over the world, especially in economically rich nations such as America, the UK and countries in Europe are now learning how to care for their hair. This information has allowed us to understand and accept the beauty of our hair. Many women wear their natural African textured hair publicly in beautiful styles, in all its glory.

CHAPTER 2

Starting a Healthy Hair Journey

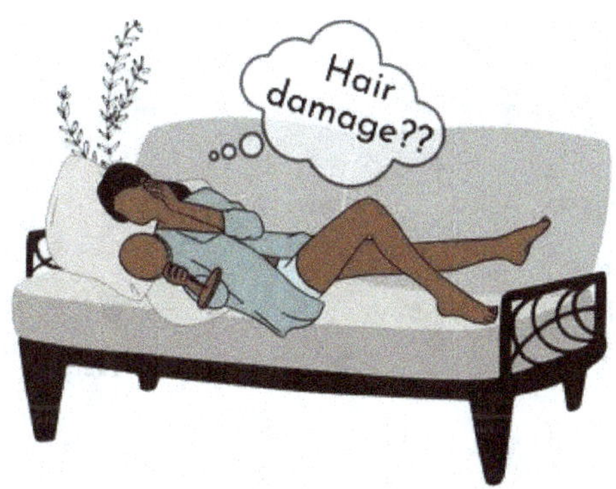

Growing your hair is a journey because it takes a long time which requires patience and commitment. So, to begin your healthy hair journey, you must start with healthy hair. Unhealthy damaged hair cannot grow. It will continuously frustrate you and slow down your progress to long healthy hair.

If your hair is damaged, your goal should be to grow out the damage and gradually cut it off, *or* cut it all off immediately (big chop) and start fresh. Remember that hair is dead and cannot be repaired, only protected from damage, and preserved.

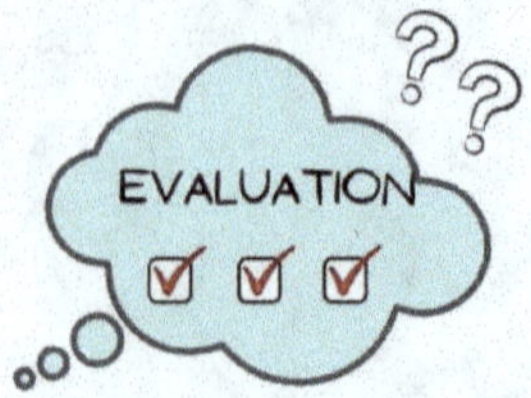

1) Damaged hair looks thin, see-through, and dry.

2) Small pieces of hair are seen during combing.

3) The ends of the hair is rough in texture.

4) Split ends are seen.

5) Hairline is missing or thin.

6) The hair is easy to break.

7) The hair is not growing.

◆ ◆ ◆

Is your hair *breaking excessively* or is it *shedding?* Let's talk about the difference between breakage and shedding.

Shedding

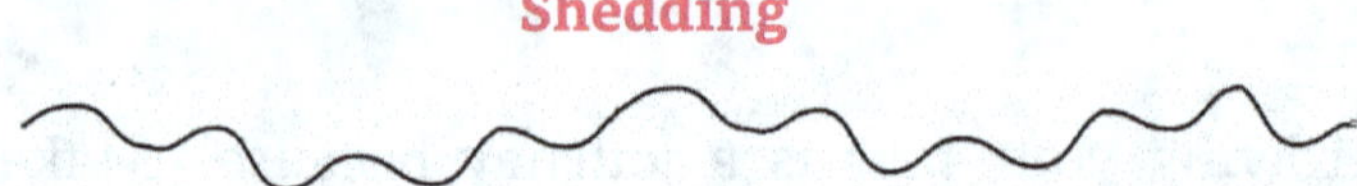

When you comb your hair, are there long strands of hair with a white dot at one end? If yes, then this is shed hair. It is normal to shed 50-100 hairs in a day. So if you keep your hair in a braided style for two months, you will notice a lot more hair on your comb because there is 60 days of shed hair.

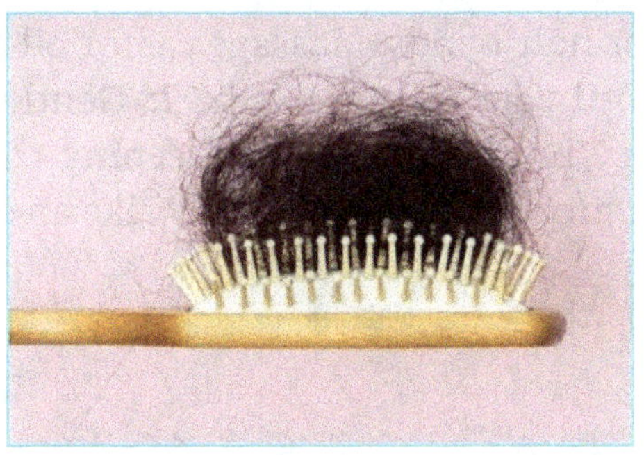

Shedding is generally not an issue to be worried about unless it is excessive. Excessive shedding can be caused by diet, severe physical or mental stress (like a divorce or loss of a family member), hormonal imbalance (post pregnancy), medication and illnesses. In such cases, a doctor should be consulted.

Breakage

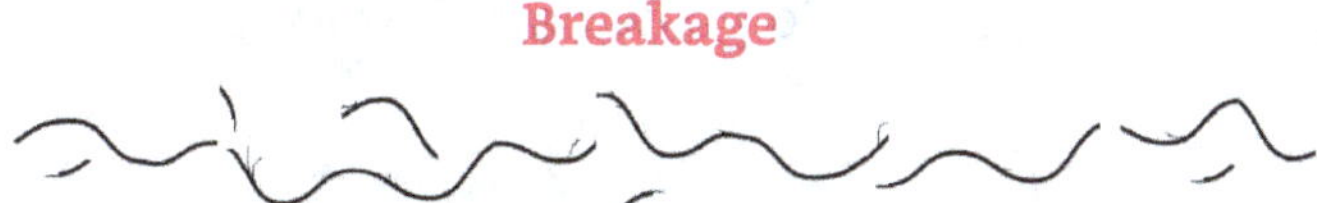

Breakage is different from shedding because it means that your hair is damaged. Weak hair is caused by careless and rough handling. If you comb your hair with small or sharp combs, it may cause tears and damage to the hair shaft (length of hair).

Every time you comb your hair, you may be inflicting small or large amounts of damage. Tearing through tangled and knotted hair also causes damage to the hair that is left behind, which leads to more breakage.

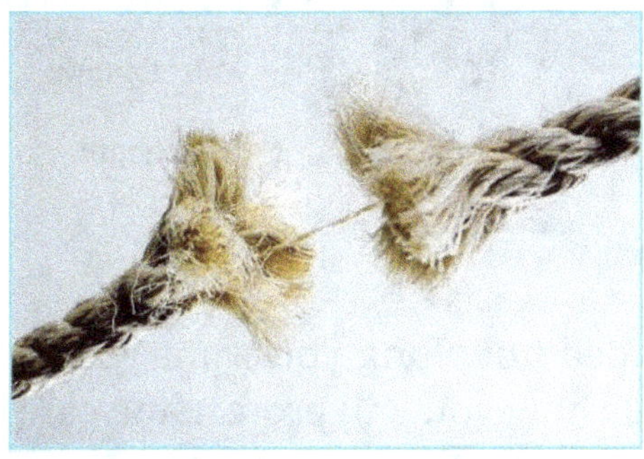

If your hairline is thin or bald, avoid braiding that area or wearing tight hairstyles or hair bands. Massage castor oil along your hairline every day until your hair grows back. Gentle detangling and handling is a very important part of keeping the hair you have grown. Your hair must be handled gently, like an egg.

If your hair is already healthy, your goal can be to grow your hair long...

Realize the *longer* you want your hair to grow, the *longer* you will have to keep your hair in protective styles, most likely 2 or more years. You will not be able to wear your own hair out, most of the time. However, don't be afraid to strive for long hair goals even if you never thought you could grow hair that long.

Pick the length you would like your hair to grow....

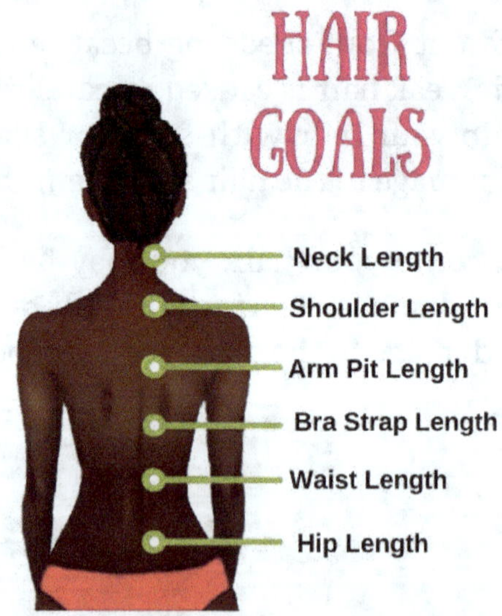

Once you've decided how long you want your hair to grow, you will need to decide how you will protect and care for your hair. As your hair grows, your methods of protecting and caring for your hair will change as you find ways that fit your lifestyle and your preferences.

CHAPTER 3

What Relaxers and Texturizers
do to Your Hair

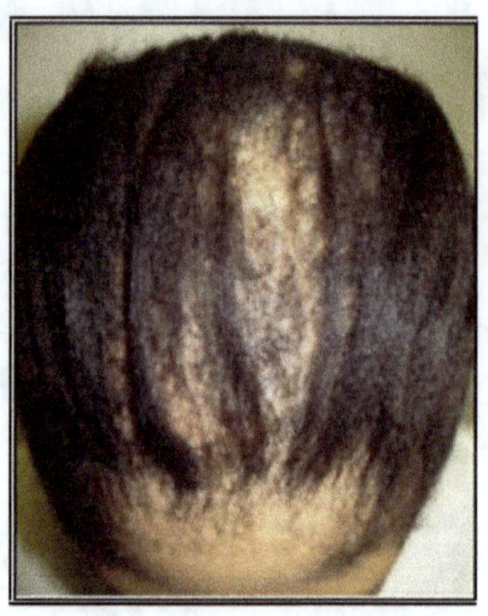

Like me, you probably remember getting your first relaxers or perms during your school years. At that time, everyone thought relaxers made our hair look straighter, which meant that it was more beautiful and easier to comb and style. Most people never thought about or understood what the chemicals did to our hair and scalp.

Without getting too technical, a single hair strand is like a tree trunk. The outer layer of the tree is what protects the tree. African textured hair represents a tree that has many bends and twists that makes those areas the weakest parts of the tree or our hair strand.

To get the hair straight...

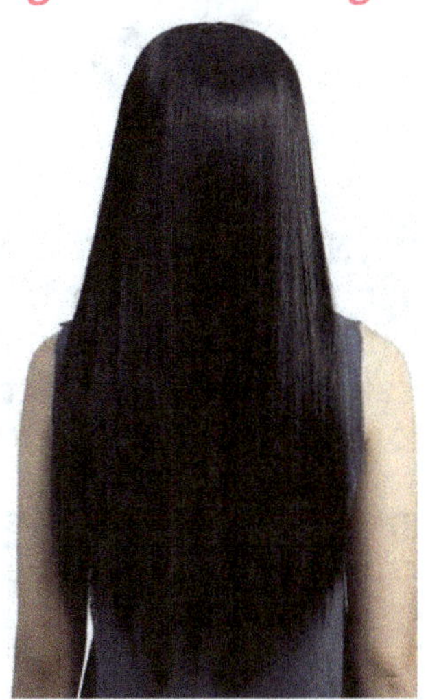

A relaxer must lift or dissolve away at the outer covering of the tree or our hair. This process also creates tears and splits to the chemically straightened bends and twists. The tree can never grow back the protective layers and can never be bent back into its strong shape again but will remain weak and damaged.

Repeated treatments done to the hair, continue to burn the hair strand and cause women to gradually lose more hair than they are growing.

Relaxers are stronger than bleach, which most ladies would never mix into a cream and put on their hair or scalp

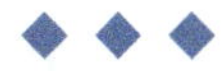

Nakuru, Kenya

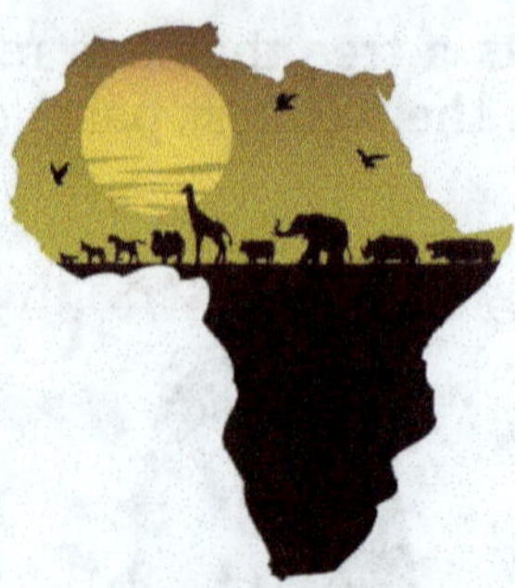

A 2006 research study in Nakuru, Kenya showed that almost 70% of relaxed haired women and girls reported experiencing burns, hair loss and color change, however almost everyone continued relaxing their hair because it was easier to manage and looked "beautiful" (Nakuru Provincial Hospital, 2006).

Relaxers have also been linked to medical issues in women of African heritage such as uterine fibroids and early puberty in young girls. For most ladies, relaxers cause thin, damaged hair that breaks off.

Most do not see hair growth and often see shorter and shorter hair, especially when relaxers are reapplied to already relaxed and damaged hair. Many are left with thinning hairlines, bald spots and sometimes permanent hair loss.

THE EXCEPTION?

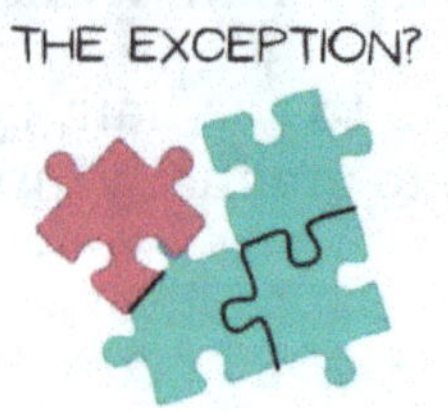

"But I know a woman who has long, beautiful, relaxed hair?"

Every woman's hair is different, but I will try to explain... These women are the EXCEPTION, meaning they *do not* represent most women with African textured hair, and yes, that includes me - and probably you too. These women already have strong hair that is generally looser textured and composed of strong elements like thicker hair strands, low porosity, and more strands (density) of hair on their heads.

I am *not* against textured or relaxed hair and I'm not telling you not to relax your hair. I want you to understand that doing so will make it much more difficult to grow your hair long.

CHAPTER 4

Trimming Your Hair

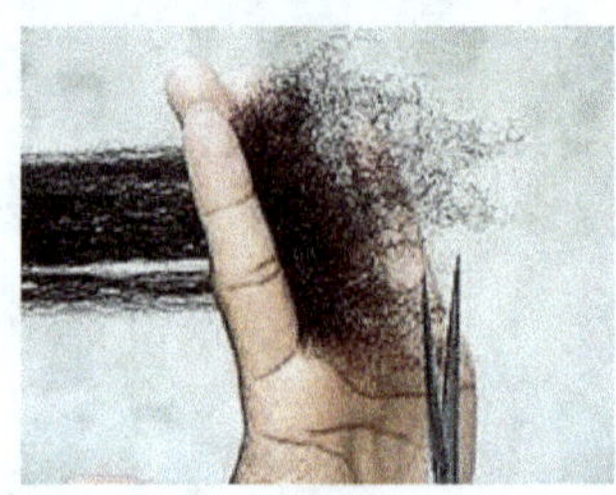

The subject of trimming is a very sensitive issue for many of us women with African textured hair. With so many of us having experienced very little hair retention, we are very fearful of cutting our hair. We are fearful that the hairdresser will cut off too much and our hair will not grow back. This is the reason why we have become attached to our hair, regardless of what it looks like.

Let's discuss why hair needs to be trimmed, how often it needs to be trimmed and how it should be trimmed.

Split Ends

The only remedy for split ends is a trim. Like the jagged end of a broken branch, split ends leave your hair damaged. This broken end will eventually create more splits and the process will continue up the hair strand.

Single Strand Knots

Single strand knots are knots at the end of your hair caused when kinky hair curls around itself. This is a common problem for type 4 hair and a reason why your hair should be kept in styles that keep your hair stretched out. Single strand knots must be trimmed off because they tangle with other hairs, creating bigger knots.

Thin Ends

Thin ends make hair look unhealthy even when it is well taken care of. It is best to trim thin ends because they are not strong enough to resist breakage from regular handling. Many hairs together are stronger than a few hairs dangling alone. These lonely danglers will continue to break off unevenly, continuing the cycle of thin ends.

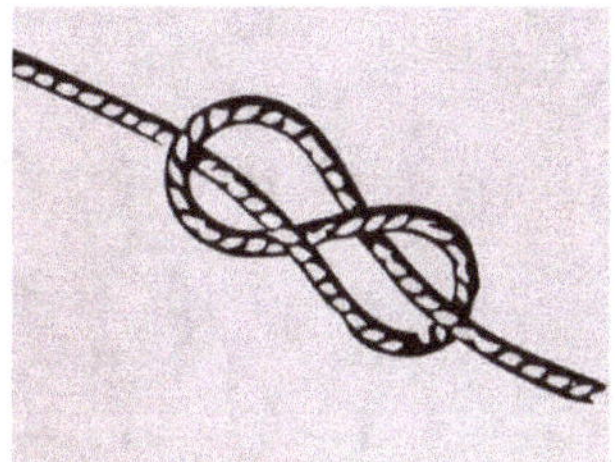

How often should you trim your hair?

Trimming is not necessary unless your hair is damaged. It really should depend on the condition of your hair. As previously mentioned, if your ends are damaged and thin, you should trim them. If your hair is healthy but there are a few single strand knots or split ends, only trim those hairs.

How should you trim your hair?

Trim your hair only when it is dry because dry hair makes a sharper cut than wet hair. Trim your hair strand straight across to avoid creating uneven ends that will lead to split ends. Use a sharp scissors that is only used for cutting your hair.

CHAPTER 5

The Science behind Your Hair Growth, Thickness and Porosity

Hair Growth Cycle

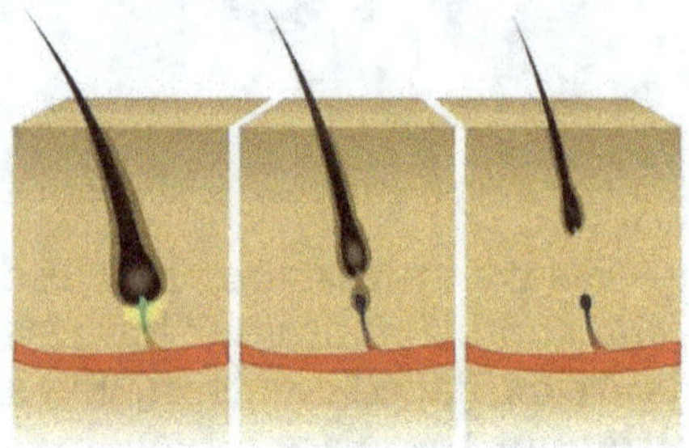

Have you ever wondered how fast your hair grows? And whether it all grows at the same rate? Or perhaps you've noticed that your hair grows more slowly than it used to? If so, you are not the only one.

When I first began to measure the rate of my hair growth, I measured four parts of my hair. The front, the left side, the right side, and the back. Within a few months I found each part had it's own growth pace. This was clearly distinguishable even by the rather basic method that I used. The back of my hair grew rapidly, the sides were about what I had expected, and the front grew the slowest.

Let me say that everyone's hair grows at it's own rate. Some are slow, and some are like *Jack and the Bean Stalk*, and grow almost an inch per month. Some months your hair will grow faster, and this process is natural. So, understand that you will experience some variation.

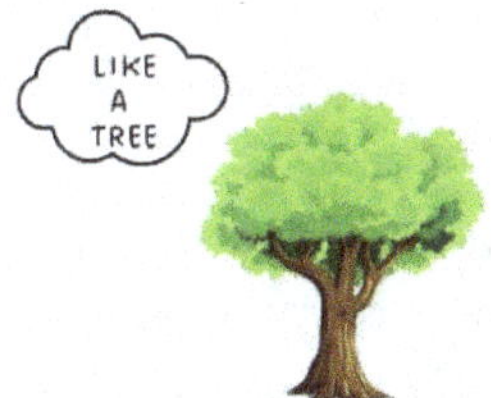

If you're trying to grow your hair long, it is important to understand the science behind how hair grows. Without getting too technical, your hair is like a tree, that tree represents your hair. A root (hair follicle) feeds the tree (hair shaft) and the tree grows. A time comes when the root stop feeding nutrients to the tree, and the tree stops growing. The root then produces a new tree which pushes out the old tree. It is the same concept with your hair.

Keep in mind that hair, like your nails, is dead. The part of the hair that is in your scalp is alive, (which is why it grows) and the part that you see on your head is dead.

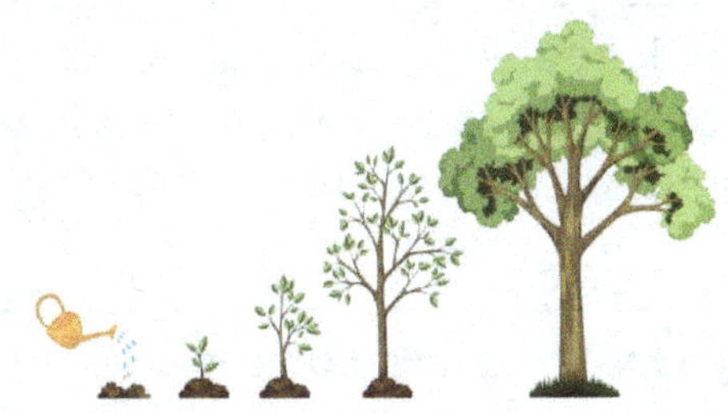

Your hair grows in three phases:

Anagen is the growing stage (tree growing) lasting from 2-6 years. 85% of your hair is growing at all times!

Catagen is the transition stage (the tree begins separating from the root) lasts from 1-2 weeks

Telogen is the shedding stage (the tree completely separates from the root and rests until new tree pushes it out) lasts from 5-6 weeks.

Some people can grow hair (the anagen stage) for 8 years! This is why you will find people with hair past their hips. On average, African textured hair grows about ½ an inch per month, which is about 6 inches a year. The average person grows hair for 5 years. That means without trimming or breakage, in 5 years, hair length should be past waist length on the average person.

Both my daughter and I have slow growing, thin, high density hair that grows at about ⅓ inch a month.

◆ ◆ ◆

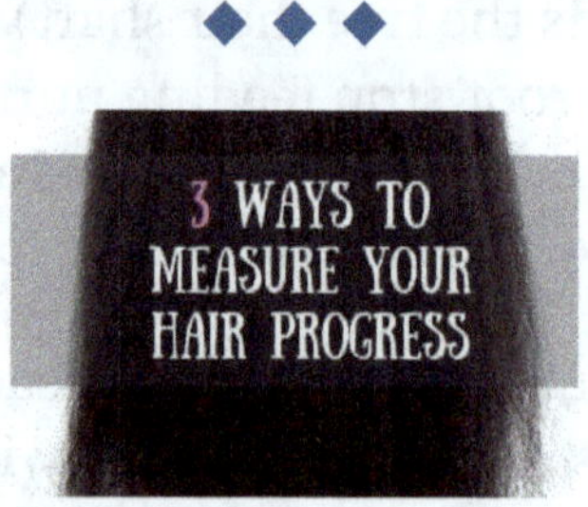

After several months to a year, there usually comes a point where you are *convinced* that your hair has stopped growing, and that it is as long as you will be able to grow it. Thankfully, you can take photographs of yourself in the mirror. This will prove to yourself that you are wrong, and that your hair *is* growing.

Take photos every three months, or at least every six months. Document how your hair grows, or those you share your journey with, will not believe that you ever struggled with your hair growth.

You can measure your hair growth casually or structured:

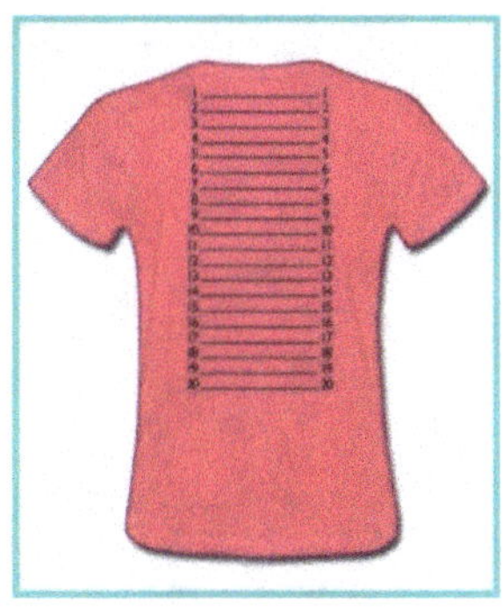

1. Your face (eyes, nose, mouth, chin, collarbone, etc) as a quick measurement.

2. A measuring tape or ruler for exact measurements.

3. A *hair length* shirt. You can buy one, or make one yourself using a plain color t-shirt and a ruler to make one inch horizontal lines from top to bottom.

CHAPTER 6

What Does Your Hair Type Mean?

HAIR TYPES

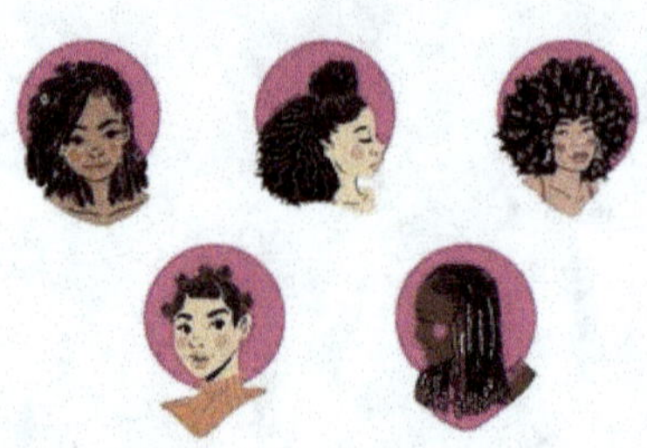

Your individual hair type consists of 3 things.

Your curl pattern
Hair thickness/density
Hair porosity

Knowing your individual hair type is important to understanding the appropriate protective styles and the products you will use in your hair care.

Before I understood about my individual hair type, I would buy every product that anyone suggested would make my hair soft, or moisturized, or strong. I would jump from one product, to the next, often disappointed as to why that product did not work on my hair.

The reason why these products did not work is because I didn't understand my individual hair type.

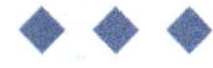

CURL PATTERN

I have 4c curl pattern. What Curl Pattern do you have?

To know your true curl pattern, look at your curls when your hair is 100% natural and wet.

Kinky textured hair is Type 4

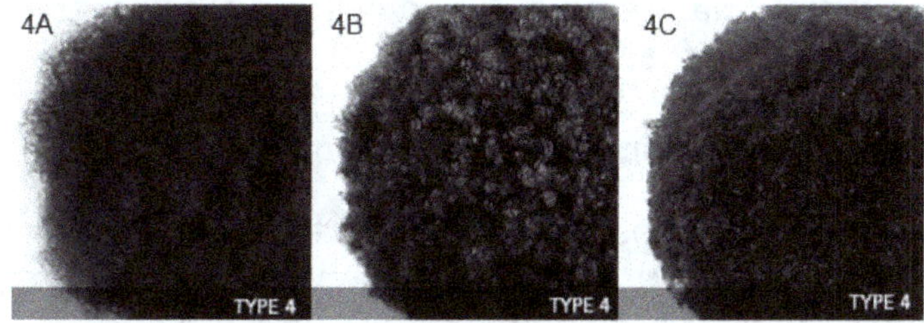

Curly textured hair is Type 3

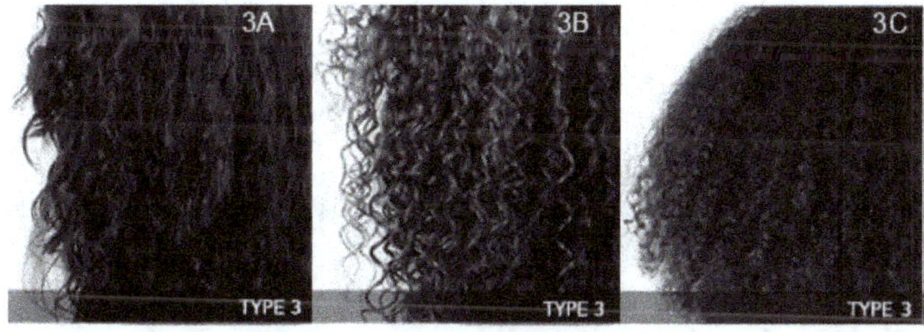

Wavy textured hair is Type 2

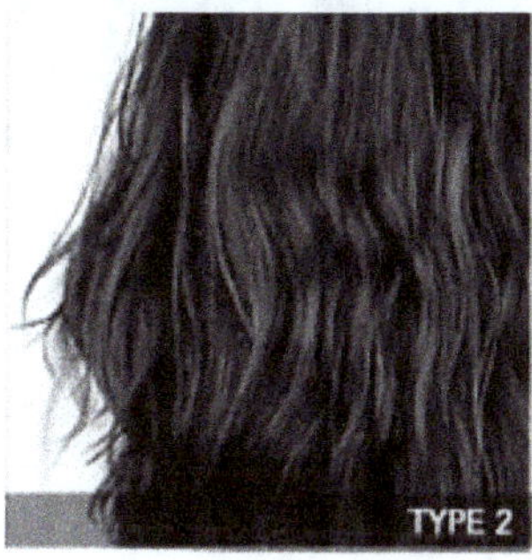

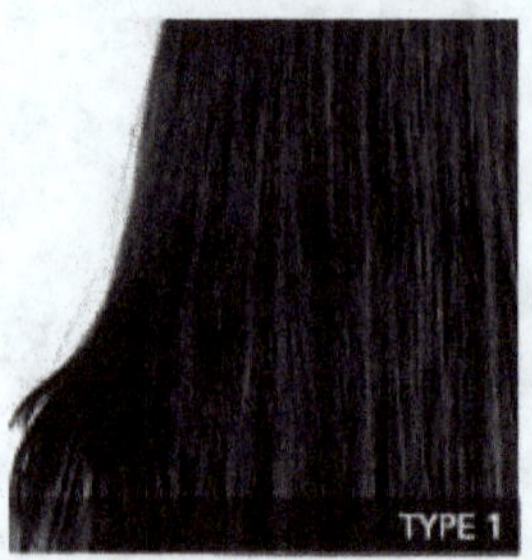

African textured hair is types 3 and 4. Type 4 hair is the most fragile, even though it feels hard. Most women have a combination of hair textures. You may have a combination of 4b and 4c. The curlier the texture, the more fragile and dry it is.

Knowing your hair type is not as important as knowing your hair thickness and porosity. Many women with the *same* hair type have *different* hair needs based on hair thickness and porosity.

HAIR THICKNESS

Your hair thickness is predetermined by your genetics. It consists of 2 things: *Hair density* and *Hair texture.* I have thin hair texture and thick hair density. Do you have thick, average, or thin hair density? And what is your hair texture? Let's find out…

HAIR DENSITY

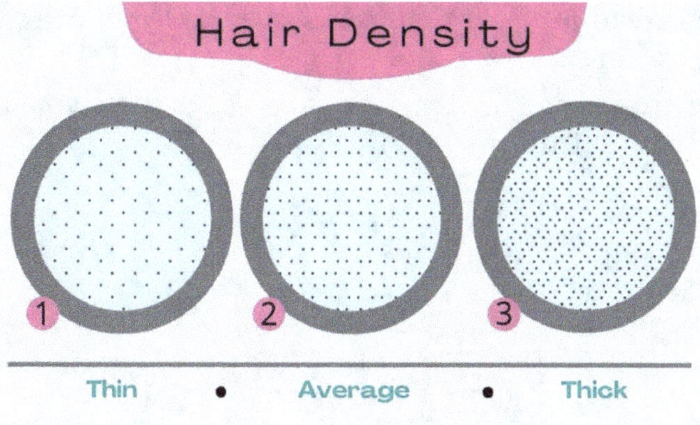

Hair Density is the number of individual strands of hair that are on your head.

Those who have thin hair density have around 90,000 hair strands on their head, average hair density is around 120,000 and those with very thick hair density have between 140,000-150,000.

HAIR TEXTURE

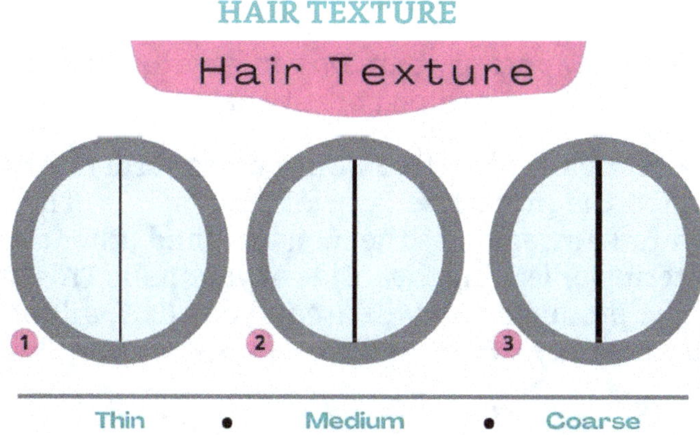

Hair Texture is the diameter (width) of the individual hair strands.

To determine your hair texture, place a single strand of your hair side by side against a piece of thread. Compare the size difference:

A) If the thread is *thicker than your hair,* then you have thin (fine) texture.

B) If the thread is *about the same size as your hair,* then you have medium texture.

C) If the thread is *thinner than your hair,* then you have thick (coarse) hair texture.

◆ ◆ ◆

HAIR POROSITY

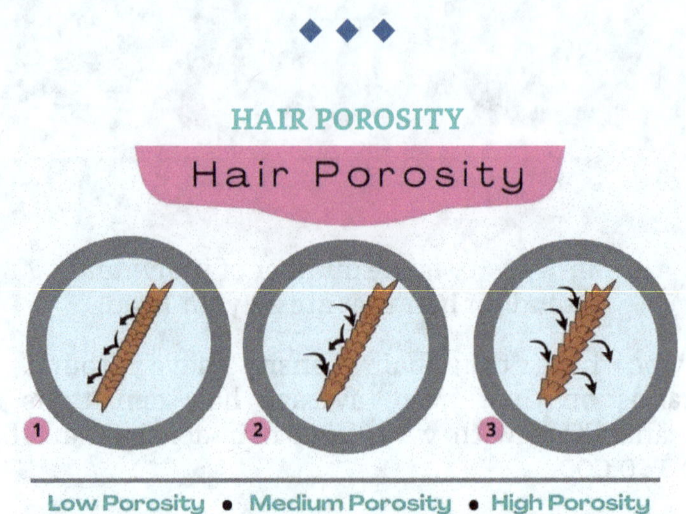

I have low porosity hair. Do you have low, medium, or high porosity hair?

Remember the bark of the tree we discussed earlier? **Hair porosity** is how lifted the protective layer of your hair is. The protective layer of your hair regulates the moisture (and other things) from either entering or leaving the inside of your hair. This means that some of the products you will use in your hair will be based on your hair's porosity.

Low Porosity (Protein Sensitive)

Hair does not relax, texturize, or color well. Hair takes a long time to dry after getting wet.

1) Test: Rub coconut oil on a small patch of your hair, if it comes stiff or hard, you have low porosity hair.

2) What this means: Your hair is in the best condition and protects itself. Therefore, you do not need heavy protein treatments. Avoid coconut oil or pure aloe vera juice

Along with your weekly washing and conditioning, your hair needs light leave in conditioners and oils such as olive, avocado or palm oils.

Medium Porosity

Hair looks and feels healthy. Hair is able to absorb oils and conditioners well.

Test: Hair feels smooth and soft after coconut oil application, Hair doesn't take too long or too short of time to dry.

What this means: Along with your weekly washing, your hair will do well with protein and moisturizing conditioning every one to two months.

High Porosity

Hair looks damaged, dry and has no shine. Hair is like a sponge and is not able to hold on to oils or conditioners.

Test: Hair feels overly greasy with coconut oil application, Hair dries very quickly after getting wet.

What this means: Along with your weekly washing, your hair needs weekly protein and moisturizing conditioners until the hair improves.

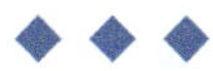

It is important that you know how your hair responds to a product that you have used on it. If your hair becomes moisturized after using a product, continue to use it. If your hair becomes dry, hard, or overly greasy after using a product, stop using that product.

*Don't force a product on your hair because it is popular
or trending. Do what is best for you and your hair.*

CHAPTER 7

Protective Styling

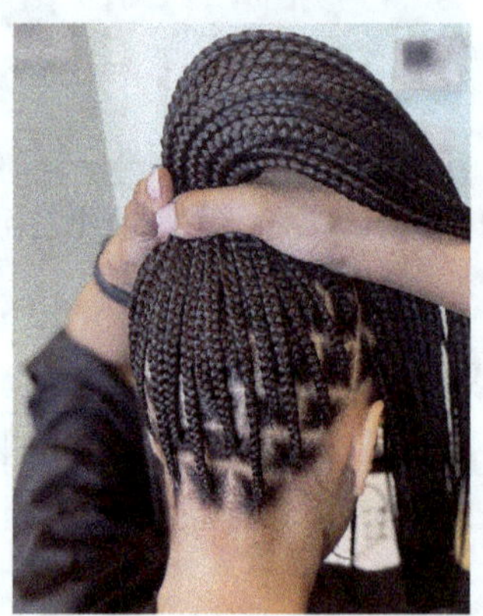

When I first went natural, I knew I would be dealing with 4c hair. I was not in any way confused about what kind of hair I had. What I struggled with was the constant dryness and breaking I experience while trying to copy the hair regimen of other ladies with different hair types than I had. I remember trying to "moisturize and seal" nightly like what I had heard others do with their hair. Instead, my hair continued to break even more, especially when I thought I was doing everything right.

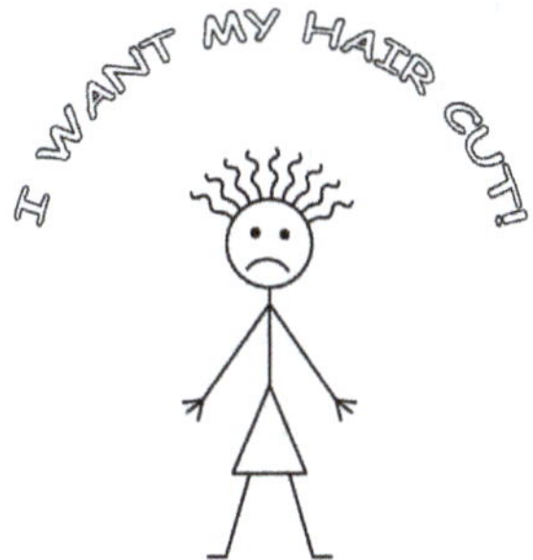

Important Lesson: Type 4 hair grows best in protective styles

I refused to accept that concept for some time because it went against what I had seen done with others who had success with growing their hair long. I tell you this to let you know that what is right for others may not be right for you.

Remember that every time you style, wash, or even touch your hair, you have a potential of damaging it. African textured hair grows best when it is not manipulated often! Even with adequate moisture, excessive manipulation will cause your hair to break.

In my opinion, it is extremely difficult for Type 4 hair to grow long without protective styling. Weekly detangling and styling while hair is loose causes significant breakage, especially in Type 4C / 4d.

Examples of protective styles (with or without hair extensions)

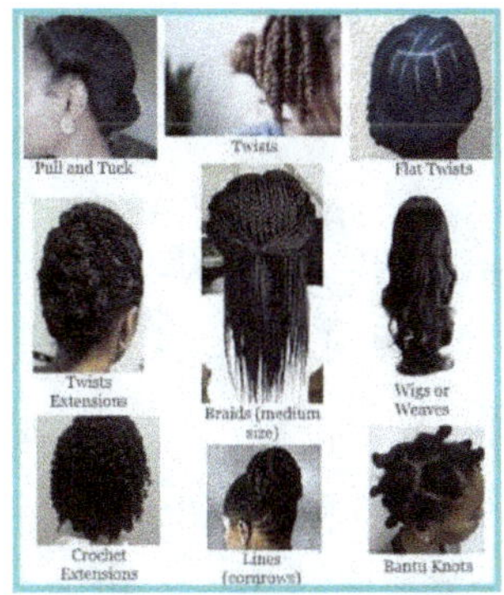

* Wigs and Weaves
* Crochet Braids
* Single Braids

* Lines or cornrows (with ends tucked in and protected)
* Twists (with ends tucked in and protected)
* Faux or fake locs

If you don't like keeping your hair in styles for an extended amount of time, then you can try styles that do not manipulate your hair in an excessive fashion. These styles are called low manipulation styles.

Examples of Low Manipulation Styles

* Braid outs and twist outs (unbraiding your braids or twists)
* Roller sets or flexi rod sets
* Roll, tuck and pin.
* Bantu knots or Bantu knot outs.

My top 5 preferred protective styling methods for growing hair long

* Yarn twists or braids
* Large or medium two strand twist with natural hair or Marley hair
* Lines (cornrows) under wigs, weaves or crochet braids
* Fake or faux locs

Top 10 Good Hair Habits to Practice!

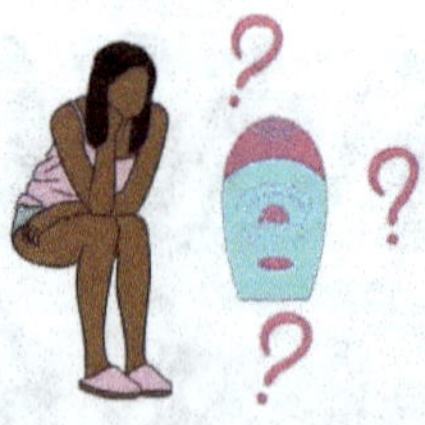

1) Gentle: Be extremely gentle with your hair!
2) Moisture: Keep hair moisturized through consistent conditioning.
3) Protect: Keep protective styles for the maximum of 2 months!

4) Wash: Shampoo and condition your hair weekly.

5) Products: Use gentle or diluted products that are not harsh.

6) Combs: Use wide-tooth combs without sharp edges.

7) Leave-in: Use leave-in conditioners.

8) Scarf: Cover your hair at night with silk or satin scarves.

9) Trim: Trim damaged ends and knots with sharp scissors for your hair only.

10: Protein Conditioner: If needed, perform a protein conditioner between long term protective styles

Top 5 Bad Hair Habits to Avoid!

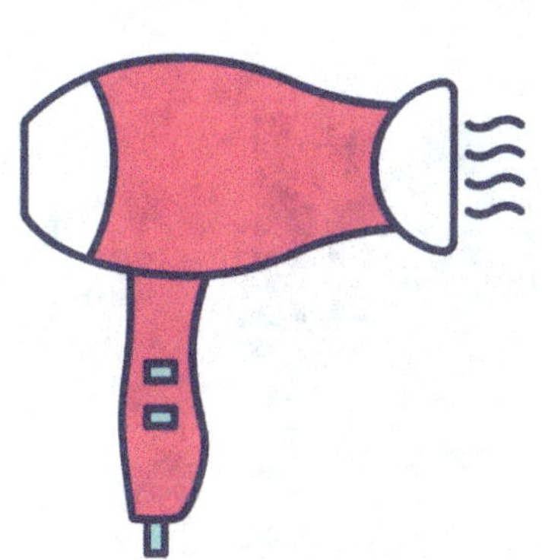

1) Limit harsh chemicals like relaxers, peroxide coloring and texturizers.

2) No tight styles! Protect your edges!

3) Limit use of direct high heat like blow drying and straightening with flat or curling iron.

4) Avoid using rubber bands or hair accessories that pull out your hair.

5) Limit excessive chlorine or salt water because they will dry your hair!

Avoid diets that eliminate certain food groups or are too low in calories –you will lose more hair than weight!

CHAPTER 8

Creating a Hair Regimen
to Retain Length

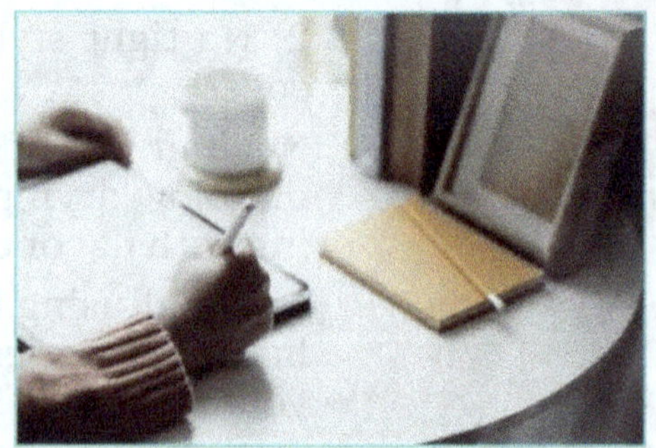

In the beginning of my hair journey, I followed a beautiful lady with waist-long relaxed hair. She had a list of all the products that she used, and how she used them. I happily wrote down the name of each product, and as soon as I got paid, I ran to the beauty supply store. I gave the store clerk the list of the 13 products I had written down, including a huge hooded dryer.

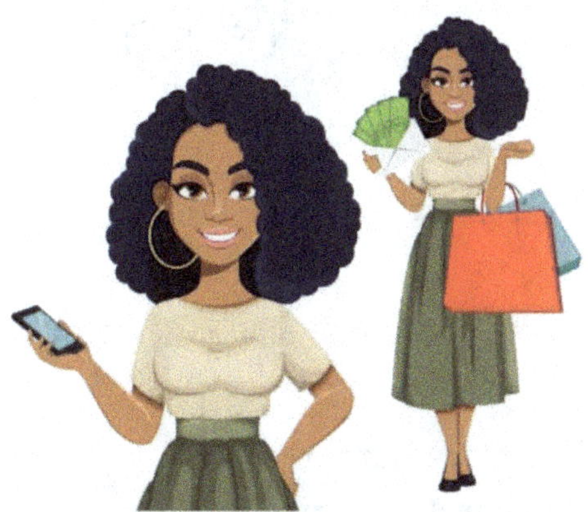

I got home and excitedly began trying the products as instructed. I spent 30 minutes under my new dryer, and I got out feeling proud of myself. After washing out the product, and applying a moisturizing treatment, some parts of my hair felt like steel wool and the other part felt like straw. I thought, well… that one will not work.

As the weeks went on, I continued to try products, thinking that my hair will get "used" to them. After a few weeks, even with additional deep conditioning, my hair started to break. It thinned so badly, that I had to cut four inches off. For slow growing hair like mine, that was over a year's worth of hair growth. The dryer is now in my closet and have not been used since that year.

Important Lesson: Keep things simple!

At the beginning of your healthy hair journey, it is important to keep things simple. Simplicity will allow you to stick with the program and allow you to easily make changes by adding or subtracting products or methods depending on how your hair responds to them.

Another thing to consider is your lifestyle. You may be a working mom, a student, or a woman with many overwhelming responsibilities. This means that you may have a lot more to do than spend a significant amount of time on your hair.

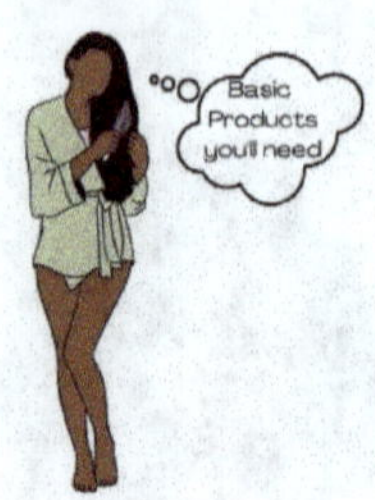

Gather the basic products that you will need for your healthy hair regimen:

1) Diluted or Sulfate free Shampoo

2) Conditioner (1 cheap, 1 quality)

3) Leave in Conditioner

4) Protein Treatment Conditioner or Henna

5) Moisturizing Treatment Conditioner

6) Natural plant oils (coconut, palm kernel, castor, avocado, and olive)

7) Glycerin and/or Rosewater

Products like coconut oil, palm kernel oil, glycerin, castor oil, rose water, olive oil, avocado oil, almond oil, avocados, eggs, and aloe vera plants are all products that are widely available at very low costs. These can be found in supermarkets, shops, or your back-yard.

Store bought products may be pricier however the tradeoff is the convenience. If these products are out of your reach, you should utilize the products that are available in your area. Don't worry about getting the fancy oils, brands or products. They don't work much better than the regular products.

Understand the Ingredients in Your Hair Products

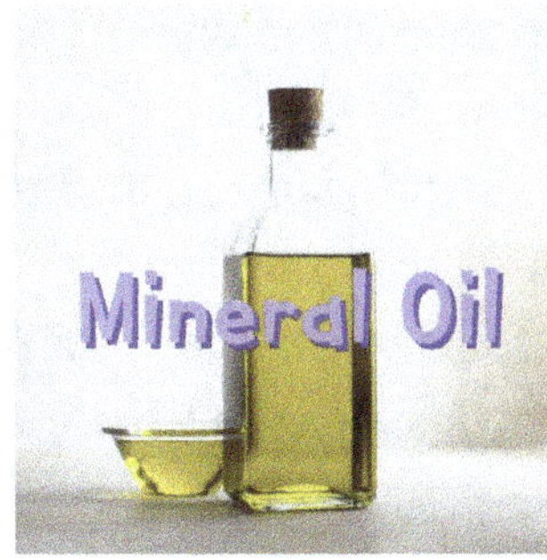

It is important to know that products do not grow your hair. Understanding what products do and how the ingredients in the products affect your hair is an important part of finding the right shampoos, conditioners etc. for your individual hair type.

Ingredients such as mineral oil, petroleum jelly, sodium lauryl / laureth sulfate (SLS), isopropyl alcohol, propylene glycol (PG), and PEG or polyethylene Glycol are some of many chemical ingredients in hair products.

Keep them in mind and know that they may negatively affect your hair growth by blocking your hair from getting enough moisture or being too harsh. If you can, try to avoid products that list them as the first 3 ingredients.

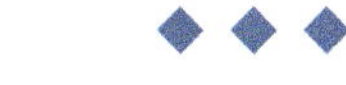

STYLING PRODUCTS FOR YOUR HAIR JOURNEY

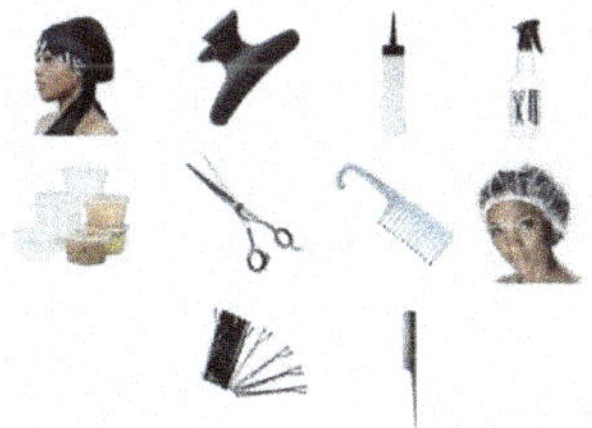

1) Hair Scarfs (silky material): To be worn at night to protect your hair.

2) Hair Clips: Use to separate hair into sections.

3) Applicator Bottles: Apply leave-in and oils to lines.

4) Plastic Containers: For conditioner or oil mixes.

5) **Hair Scissors:** Sharp scissors used for your hair only.

6) **Wide Tooth Comb:** For detangling.

7) **Hair Pins:** For styling updos or roll and tucks.

8) **Plastic caps:** Use for deep conditioning.

9) **Rat Tail Comb:** Use for parting hair and lines.

10) **Spray Bottles:** Spray leave-in conditioners and oils.

CHAPTER 9

Hair Regimen Examples (Part 1)

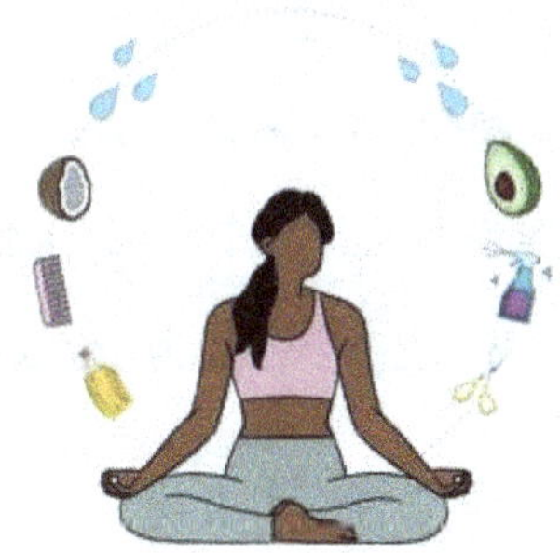

The hair regimen examples below are simple. They will allow you to easily wash, moisturize and style your hair without too much manipulation. Keep in mind that the process of installing long term protective styles can be very damaging to your hair. Pulling, blow drying, rough combing, and ripping through tangled hair is a major reason for hair not growing.

Important Lesson: Rough handling during hair styling will cause you to lose the inches you have grown.

For long term protective styles (1-2) months, perform a protein treatment or henna (if needed) and a moisturizing treatment before installing your style.

● ● ●

Twists, Flat Twists, Cornrows or Lines, Wigs

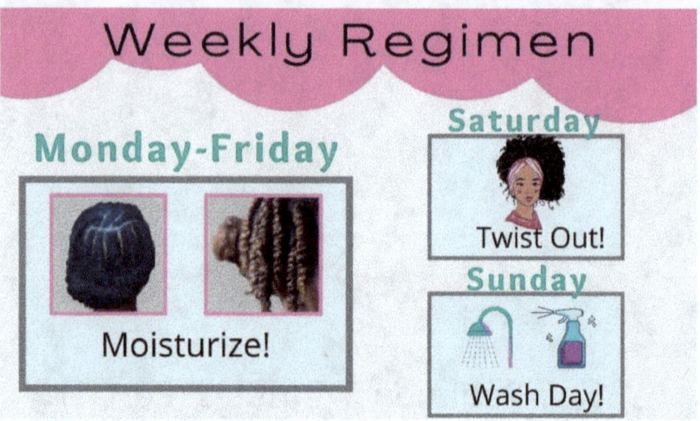

Twists, cornrows (lines), crochet braids and wigs work well for both Type 3 and Type 4 hair.

Monday-Friday : Spray hair with leave-in conditioner and oils.

Saturday or Monthly: Twist-out or Braid-out. Pineapple at night.

Sunday or Monthly: Wash, Condition and Re-Style.

Braids or twists with Extensions, Fake locs

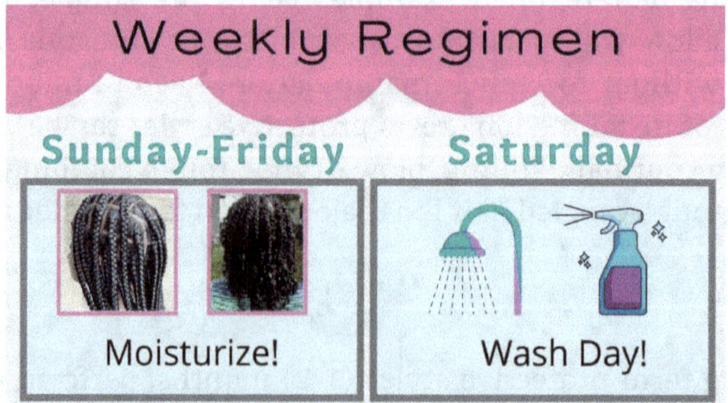

If you have Type 4 hair, braids and twists are the easiest protective style to maintain.

Sunday-Friday: Spray hair with leave-in conditioner and oils.

Saturday or monthly: Wash, condition, and leave-ins.

Nightly: Wrap hair with silk scarf.

It is best to keep your hair in protective styles that stretches out your curls to avoid knots and tangles. Be sure the braid sections are medium sized and not too small, too heavy, or too tight.

Buns, Roll and Tucks

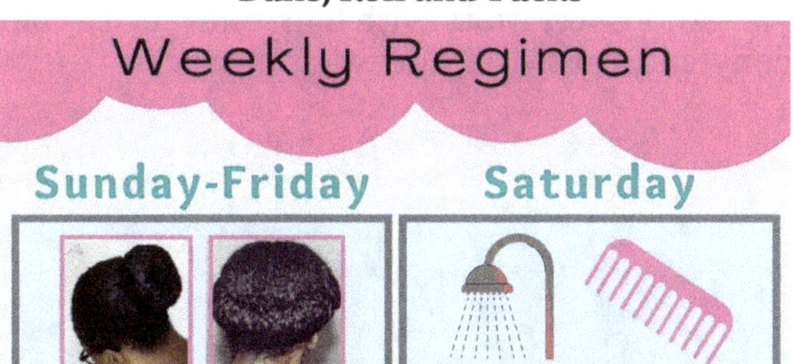

High buns, low buns, and side buns are great options for Type 3 and 4a hair.

Sunday-Friday: Style hair, moisturize and seal nightly. Wrap hair at night.

Saturday or Monthly: Shampoo, condition, moisturize and re-style.

Nightly: Wrap hair with silk scarf.

Buns should be alternated to reduce breakage from keeping your bun in the same spot. Hair should be moisturized and sealed nightly, then placed into a high ponytail on top of your head. Wrap a scarf around your head with the curls sticking out at the top, like a pineapple. Cover your pillow with a silky material if you don't have a satin or silk pillowcase. You can also insert your pillow into an old silky shirt.

In the morning, pass a brush lightly over the top of your hair to smooth it into a bun. Do not comb your entire head of hair, only the perimeter, so your bun looks neat. Tuck in the ends of your hair to keep it protected. If your hair is short, you can use braided hair extensions that match your hair type, or a rolled-up sock, to make your bun look bigger.

If you have short Type 3 hair, it is best to keep the ends of your hair in protective styles with medium sized braids or "wash and go's" until your hair gets to your shoulders. As your hair gets longer, you will have more versatility with hairstyles such as buns, large, braided ponytails, flat twists, and wrap and tucks.

CHAPTER 10

Hair Regimen Examples
(Part 2- Simple)

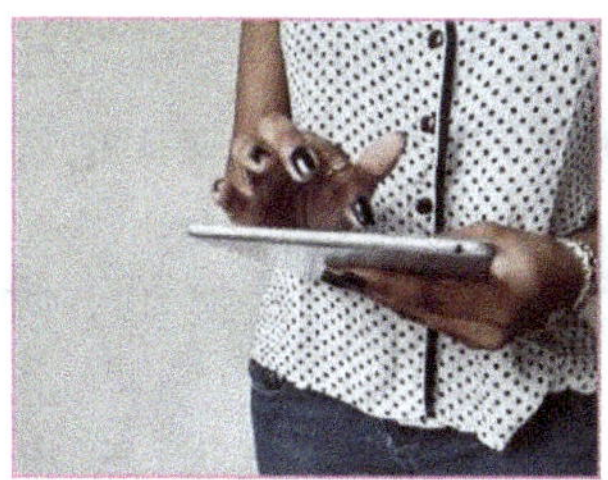

Trying to grow your hair with your hectic, jam-packed schedule can feel like trying to swim upstream. While you dutifully fit in those morning routines, meetings, errands, studying and several stops to connect with your friends and loved ones, the massive effort it takes to take care of your hair doesn't always seem worth it.

That is why when you are trying to grow your hair, you should keep things very simple. I know that for some ladies, a lengthy hair routine can be unrealistic. I have designed three amazingly simple regimens that will keep you on track - without wasting your precious time.

SIMPLE BRAID REGIMEN
(for busy students)

What you'll need (You may have some of these at home).

1) Any shampoo: Sulfate free, or diluted shampoo.

2) Any conditioner: For conditioning and detangling.

3) Deep conditioner: Giovanni, ORS, African's Best or your pre-ferred brand.

4) Oils: Olive or coconut oil, or melted shea butter.

5) Scalp Treatment: Sulfa-8 for scalp or Virgin Hair Fertilzer (optional).

BRAIDS, TWISTS, OR FAUX LOCKS
(with your own hair, extensions, or crochet)

Keep your hair in crochet or braids (medium sized). 1-2 months at a time. Perform your deep conditioning (protein and moisturizing) treatment in between styling. Do this for 2-3 years while in school. It is the easiest way to grow your hair as a busy student.

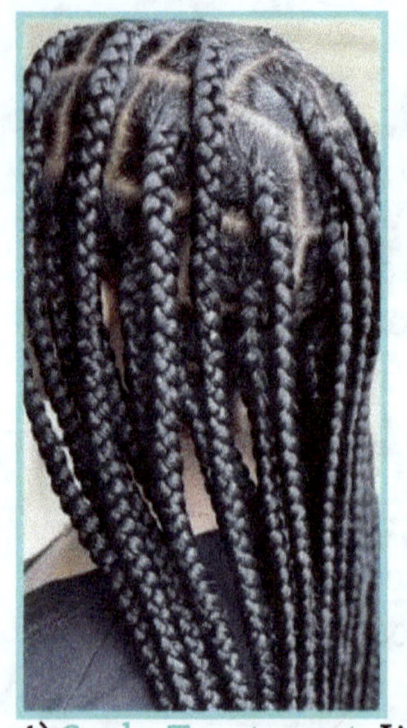

1) Prep and Style: Gently wash and detangle your hair yourself before going to the salon. Do not blow dry your hair. Avoid braiding your hairline or tight braids.

2) Weekly Wash: Once a week, wash your hair and scalp while in the braids or twists, with diluted shampoo and your cheap conditioner.

3) Leave-in: After your hair is almost dry, spray your leave-in conditioner mixed with your oils, on the parts where your hair is.

4) Scalp Treatment: When your hair is completely dry, apply Sulfa-8 to your scalp.

Once your hair has grown to your desired length, you may use your own hair for braids and twists, and follow the same routine.

Style your own hair on special occasions, so that you may enjoy your progress as it grows.

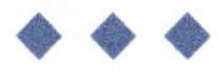

TINY LITTLE AFRO REGIMEN

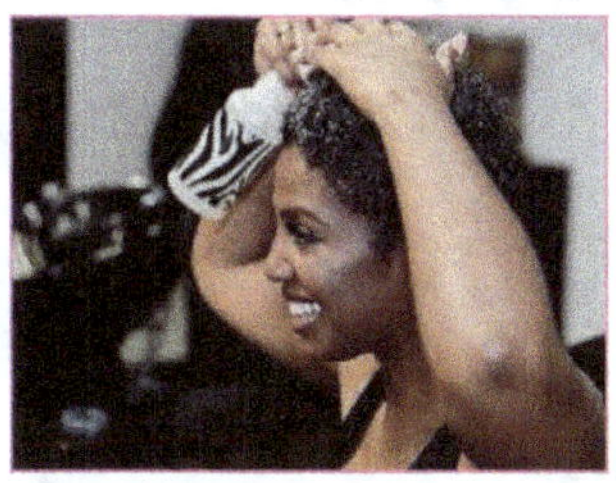

From 0-6 months:

1) Massage your scalp weekly right before washing.

2) Shampoo and condition your little afro. After a few months, your hair will be long enough to start detangling with conditioner.

3) When your hair is almost dry, apply your leave-in conditioner and favorite oils. (I use ORS or Africa's Best)

4) After your hair is completely dry, apply Sulfa-8 to your scalp. Sulfa-8 is great at preventing itching and dandruff.

5) Cover your hair with a satin or silk scarf every night.

6) In the morning, apply your leave-in and gently comb out your Afro.

7) Take photos every 1-2 months, on your wash day.

SIMPLE WIG REGIMEN

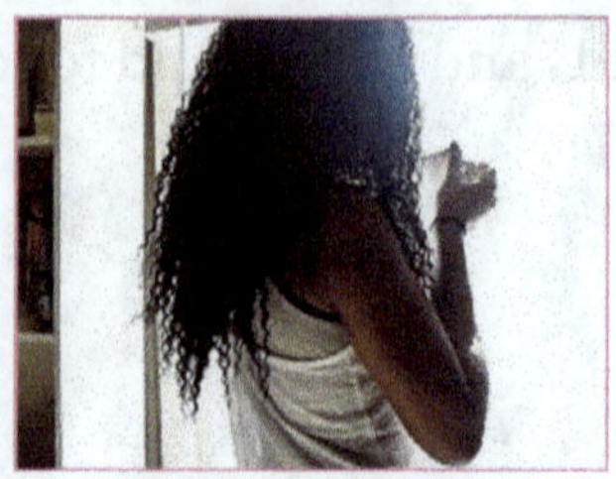

Wigs are a great option because you can change styles while having full access to your hair underneath.

SAMPLE PRODUCTS

(Use your preferred products)

Mane'n Tail Shampoo

Mane'n Tail Conditioner

Giovanni Leave-in Conditioner

Coconut Oil, Olive Oil or Melted Shea Butter

Aphogee 2 minute Reconstructor

Aphogee Moisturizing Treatment

Sulfa-8

Applicator bottles (2). One for your diluted shampoo mixture, the other for your conditioner/oil mixture.

Every 1-2 months:

1) Detangle: Gently detangle your hair with Mane'n Tail conditioner.

2) Shampoo: Shampoo your hair with Mane'n Tail Shampoo.

3) Protein Conditioner: Apply your protein treatment with Aphogee 2 minute Reconstructor

4) Moisturizing Treatment: Apply Aphogee Balancing Moisturizer for 30 minutes.

5) Leave-in Conditioner and oils: Apply when hair is almost dry.

6) Style: Re-do your cornrows while hair is still damp. Fold over

the ends of your cornrows, apply extra conditioner and oils, then tuck them underneath. Avoid exposing the ends of your hair to friction from your wigs.

7) Scalp: Apply Sulfa-8 to your scalp once your hair is completely dry.

Weekly

1) Shampoo and Condition: Using diluted shampoo and conditioner using applicator bottles.

2) Washing: Apply shampoo mixture to your scalp and cornrows. Massage each cornrow in a circular motion as your go from front to back.

3) Rinsing: Rinse off and let hair dry.

4) Leave-in: Apply diluted leave-in conditioner.

Daily

Wear your hair bonnet or scarf nightly. A silk pillowcase in place of a scarf or bonnet is another option.

ALLERGY WARNING: Product examples may contain ingredients that you may be allergic to. Please perform a patch test before committing to using any product examples in this guide.

CHAPTER 11

Step by Step Guide on how to Wash African Textured Hair

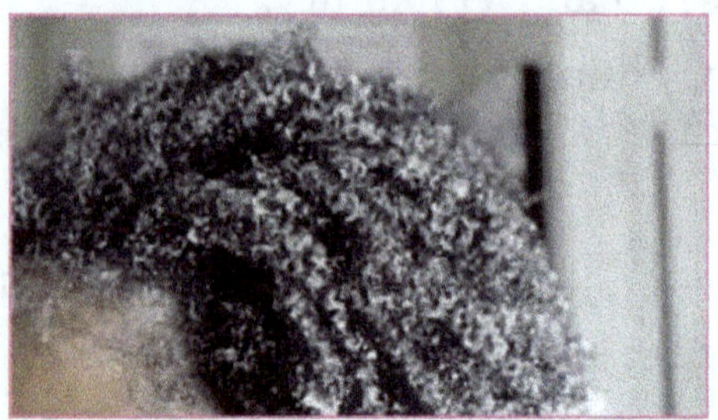

Moisturizing African textured hair is one of the most important aspects of growing long hair. To provide proper moisture, hair needs water. Oils and creams cannot replace water. Just as water is important to the body, water is also important to keeping your hair in a healthy condition.

Unfortunately, this is the area where most fail in their journey to having long hair. Bad habits of not washing or moisturizing our hair often tend to stay with us even after we have made the decision to grow our hair long and practice healthy hair care habits.

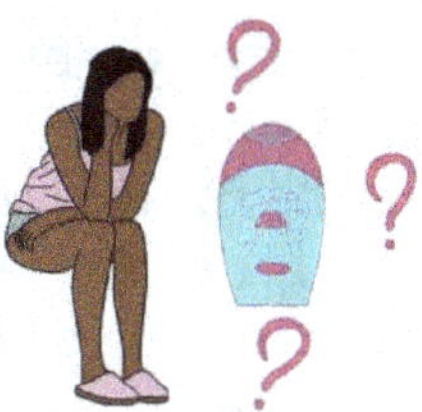

To avoid wasting years and seeing continuous breakage and no growth beyond a certain point, make the commitment to wash and moisturize your hair as much as you practice protective styling. The first thing you must always keep in mind is that African textured hair is the most fragile and gentle handling must be practiced when washing your hair. Now let's discuss this in detail...

How often should you wash your hair?

Some women wash their hair three times a week, some every day. Different women may require different hair care and eventually you will find a routine that suits you best. However, to start, wash your hair once a week.

How should you wash your hair?

You must be very gentle with your hair, especially while it is wet. Wet hair can break without *hearing* it break. Use the pads of your fingertips to massage your scalp in a circular motion while washing. Avoid using your nails which can create small tears that can lead to scalp problems.

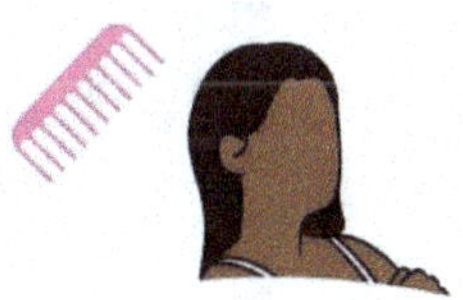

Step 1: Detangling

Only wash your hair after it has been detangled. Section your hair into 6-12 big twists or plaits and apply a cheap conditioner to each twist. Your hair becomes more elastic when it is wet, so this reduces the chance of your hair tangling and breaking.

Use a wide tooth comb to gently detangle your hair from tip (bottom) to root (top). This helps to prevent tangles. Retwist your hair after each section has been detangled. If you find knots or tangling, stop and gently pull the tangled and knotted hairs apart with your fingers. If you are unable to remove a knotted strand, you must cut it off with your hair scissors.

Side Note: You can also use your fingers to detangle your hair by separating your hair into small sections, while gently pulling through for shed hair. This is called finger detangling. Many ladies with natural 4c hair type, have had success growing their hair to waist length, by using their fingers alone to detangle their hair and never a comb.

Step 2: Shampoo

Apply shampoo to your scalp and use your fingertips to massage the dirt off your scalp in a circular motion. Gently smooth the shampoo down the hair, section by section, then rinse thoroughly.

Step 3: Conditioning

Apply your quality conditioner down your twists and leave it in for 5-10 minutes. Rinse off your twists in cool water (this helps your hair to stay moisturized).

Step 4: Drying

Use a towel to gently squeeze the water from each twist. Then, apply an old shirt to cover your hair instead of wrapping the heavy towel around your fragile hair strands.

Step 5: Leave-in conditioner

Leave-in conditioners help your hair to be soft and flexible for styling. After your hair is almost dry (around 75%), apply your leave-in conditioner to each twist and style your hair in your desired protective or low manipulation hair style.

Co-Washing and Oil Rinsing

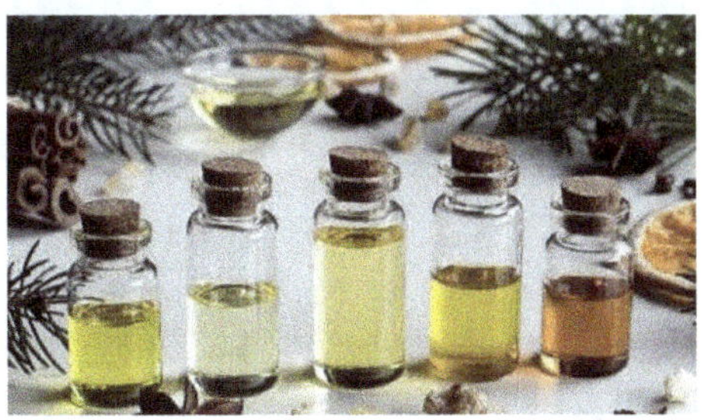

If you find that your hair is dry in between washes, use conditioner only to wash your hair, rinse, and then when your hair is 75% dry, apply your leave-in conditioner or oils. This is called conditioner washing, or co-wash.

Alternatively, you can use your oils to do an oil rinse by smoothing the oil mixture through your hair, rinse, and then when your hair is 75% dry, apply your leave-in conditioner or oils.

Co-washing and oil-rinsing are not necessary to do as long as your hair stays moisturized with your regular hair care regimen.

Washing Your Hair in Braids, Twists and other Long-Term Styles

If your hair is in a long-term protective style, you should also wash and condition your hair weekly while it is in the protective style. To do this, use your applicator bottles with diluted shampoo and conditioners, gently rub your scalp and hair, rinse, dry to 75%. Using your applicator bottles, apply your leave-in conditioner or oil mix to your lines or cornrows.

CHAPTER 12

Deep Conditioning Treatments

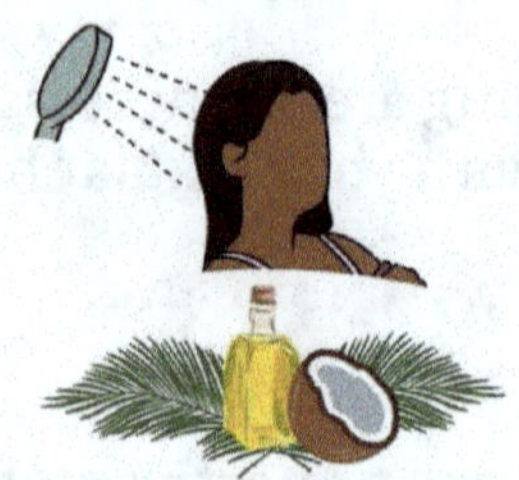

The two deep conditioning treatments that are important to a healthy hair care regimen are protein deep conditioners and moisturizing deep conditioners. Protein deep conditioners keep your hair strong and moisturizing deep conditioners keep your hair soft and moisturized.

Too many protein treatments can cause your hair to become hard and too many moisturizing treatments can cause your hair to become too soft. Both situations can cause your hair to break, so before doing either deep conditioning treatment, you will need to check the condition of your hair first.

Stretch Test:

To do this, get three to four strands of shed wet hair (after wash-

1) If your hair does not stretch but breaks, then your hair needs a moisturizing deep conditioning treatment.

2) If your hair stretches to 20-30% and stays stretched, then your hair needs a protein deep conditioning treatment.

3) If your hair stretches and then comes back to normal, then your hair is in good condition and does not need a protein or moisturizing deep conditioning treatment.

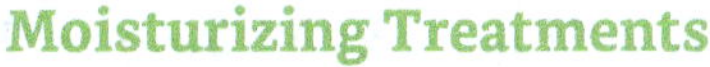

Moisturizing Treatments

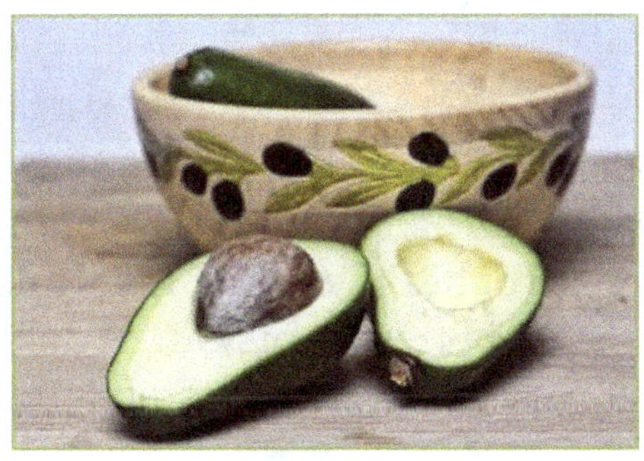

Moisturizing deep conditioners do not contain protein. This is a special treatment that can be done weekly, monthly or every two months if you are wearing a long-term protective style. This treatment can also be done if the hair feels extra dry, hard, or brittle and should help reduce breakage.

This treatment replaces step 3 of the "How should you wash your hair" section. Depending on the moisturizing deep conditioner you use, you will need to follow the specific direction given on the product. To avoid over moisturizing your hair, be sure not to go beyond the time instructed or 30 minutes. Continue with Steps 4 and 5.

Steam Treatments

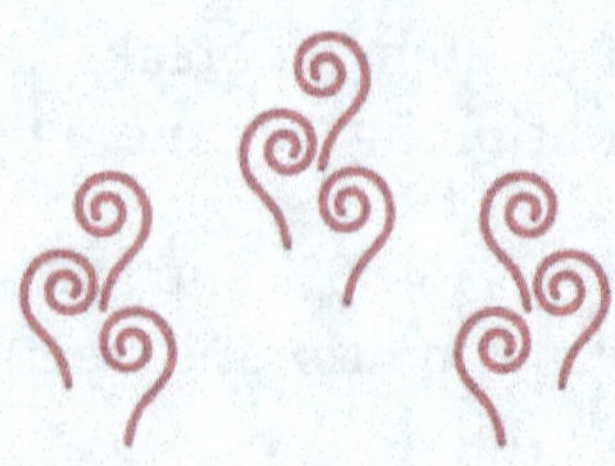

This is the best way to get moisture into dry hair. This is especially great in between long-term protective styles and after a protein treatment. This treatment is usually done at the beauty salon and replaces the hooded dryer.

Protein Treatments

Your hair is 91% protein. Deep protein conditioners add protein to the hair to help weak hair become temporarily stronger and maintain the strength of healthy hair. It is useful if you have thin or damaged hair. Protein treatments can be done every one-two month if your hair feels weak, mushy, or too soft.

A protein treatment needs to be done on thoroughly shampooed hair. The protein works more efficiently when the hair is without oil, butters, or conditioner. Depending on the protein deep conditioner you use, you will need to follow the specific directions given on the product.

Continue with Steps 4 and 5 of the "How should you wash your hair" section. Always follow a protein conditioner with a moisturizing deep conditioner.

How to Deep Condition Your Hair at Home

For home deep conditioning, smooth the conditioner down to the ends of your hair, cover your hair with a plastic cap then cover again with several scarves to keep your body heat in the cap. Keep on for 30 minutes or follow the directions given on the product you are using.

Something to consider...

Not every hair responds well to protein conditioners or proteins of any kind. For example, coconut oil, silk and keratin protein conditioners are some products containing protein that are often used by some in their healthy hair regimen. However, there are women like me, or maybe even you, whose hair becomes dry, hard, and brittle when these products are used on our hair.

Henna and aloe vera can also cause these issues. If you have tried these products and they make your hair hard, you may try to reduce the amounts to half or remove them altogether from your hair products.

CHAPTER 13

Finding the Right Hairdresser

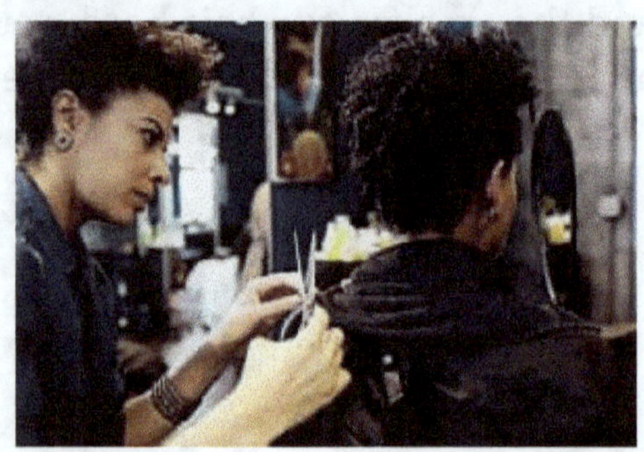

Try to find hairdressers that have been educated on natural hair and are willing to assist you in your hair care needs.

It is important that when you go to a hairdresser that you bring your personal hair products so that she will use them in your hair. If she does not have experience in caring for natural hair, politely explain that you are trying to grow your hair long and that you want your hair to be detangled with your conditioner and combed very gently starting from the ends.

Explain that you want your tangles and knots removed gently with her fingers and not ripped through with a comb. You can also explain that you do not want your hair blow dried and if you do, on a low or medium heat, gently with the comb attachment. Keep reminding your hairdresser to keep your braids or twists loose and not too tight to avoid your hair from thinning. Your hairline should not be braided as to avoid a bald hairline.

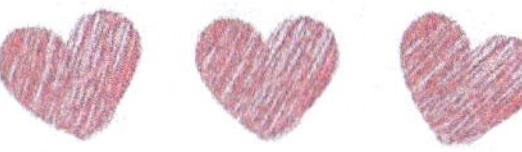

If a stylist does not understand after you have tried explaining, do not be afraid to refer her or him to this book. Soon there will be more and more natural hair ladies coming to her salon and it will be in her or his financial benefit to learn about taking care of natural hair.

If you are not receiving the services you have requested, apologize, and thank your hairdresser, get up and go to another place. If you cannot find a suitable stylist, learn to do your own hair. Do not risk damaging your healthy hair because you are afraid to speak up.

CHAPTER 14

Healthy Body for Healthy Hair

Exercise

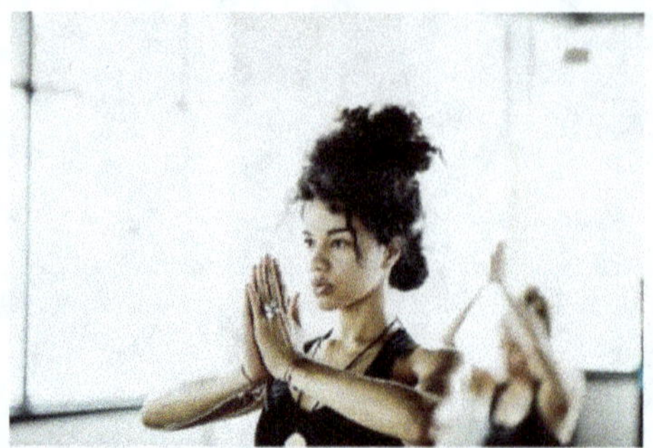

Exercise is not only important to keeping your body healthy; it is the best available anti-aging, hair growth system available to us for free, it is best to take advantage of the benefits it provides. Exercise is also one of the most underrated systems for growing your hair to its full potential.

My hair grows slowly, at about 1/3 of an inch per month. With exercise, my hair growth increases to ½ of an inch per month. Exercise works.

Diet

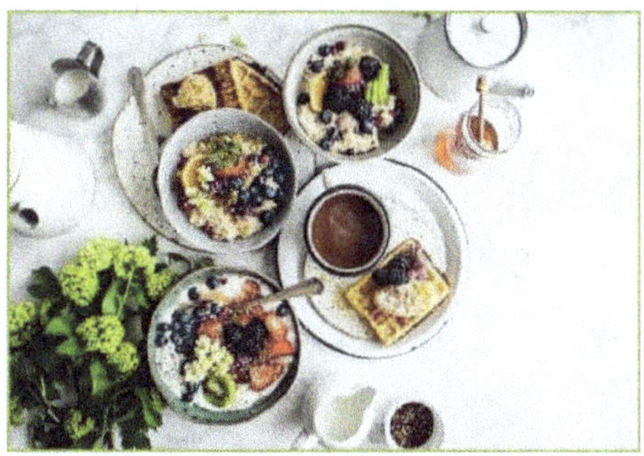

Your diet can affect how your hair grows. Remember that your hair is dead. Your body does not care about growing your hair as much as it cares about taking care of the rest of your body. Your body will sacrifice your hair and nails to provide nutrients to your body first.

Be sure that your diet is not lacking in protein (beans, greens, and legumes), fruits, vegetables, whole grains (maize, etc), dairy (milk, eggs) and water. You can choose to take a multivitamin if your diet is deficient, but it is not necessary with an already balanced diet.

Stress

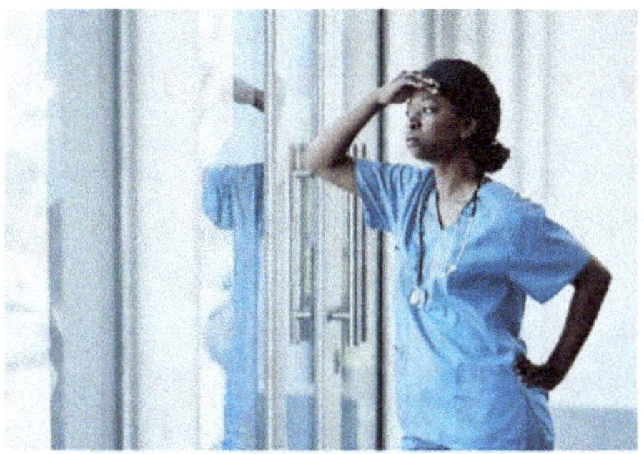

When girls and women go through stressful situations such as losing a family member, a divorce, or severe physical stress (illness) and emotional stressors, they can lose their hair. The body sends a signal to the hair follicles and tells them to stop growing. This can cause massive shedding, thinning, and hair coming out in clumps.

If you have excessive hair loss, evaluate your current situation, and see if you know what is causing it. It may require you to see your doctor who can give you suggestions on how to treat your hair loss.

Hormonal Changes

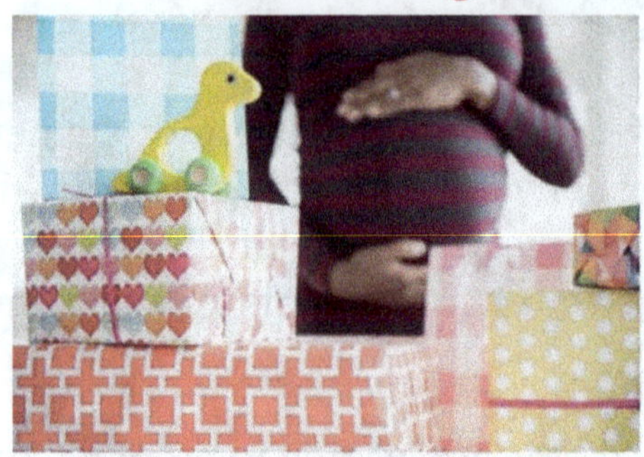

Women can experience hair growth during pregnancy and hair loss after pregnancy. This is not permanent, and the hair will grow back, even if it seems traumatizing at the time. It is best to style your hair in braids or twists, so you are not excessively manipulating your hair. Men also experience hair loss due to hormonal changes.

Hair Potions, Lotions and Miracle Hair Growth Serums

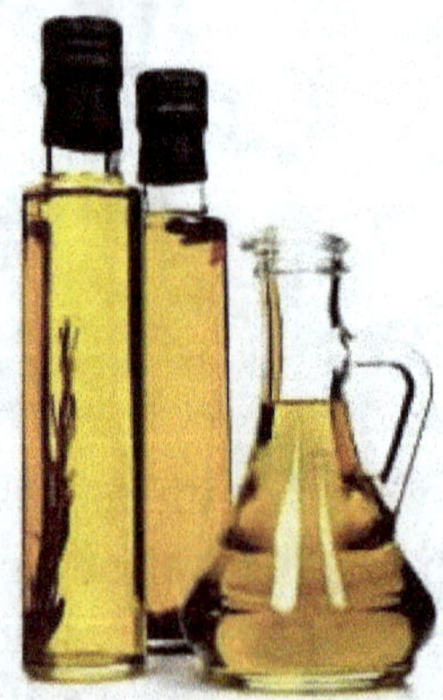

Be very cautious when you hear of a product that can grow your hair *very fast.* Remember that hair takes a long time to grow, ½ an inch per month on average. People everywhere are aware of the struggles of retaining hair that African textured hair women and girls have, they take advantage of this and try to scam the uninformed and innocent out of their hard-earned cash.

There are Facebook ads, with fake reviews from people testifying that the product worked for their hair. There is no lotion or potion out there that can grow your hair *very fast*.

Please, avoid these scams. If it is too good to
be true, it is probably a scam.

Long, healthy hair takes time and dedication with healthy hair care practices. Remember your hair is already growing; the best results come from maximizing your ability to keep the hair that is growing.

Hair growth medication like Biotin works on and increases the anagen phase of the hair growth cycle. Do understand that everything has its side effects. It has worked wonders for many women, but some have also experienced massive shedding, thinning and acne from using it.

CHAPTER 15

Guide to Growing an African Textured Child's Hair Long

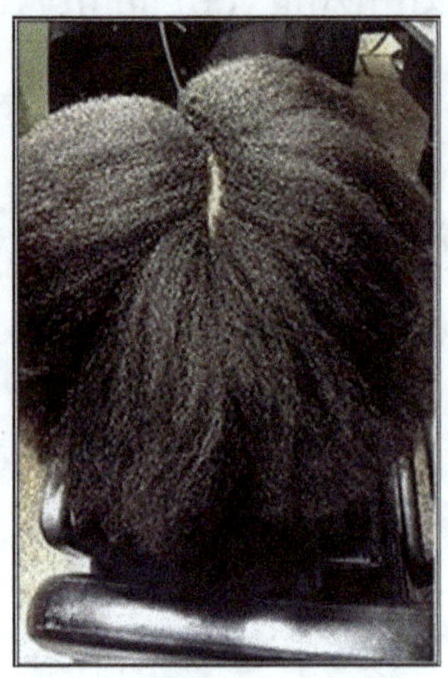

A little girl needs a simple hair regimen so that she will develop a love for her hair. Her hair regimen should allow her the freedom to have fun, play, or swim like all children love to do.

Keep things simple with long term protective styles and be sure to follow all the rules in the "Do's and Don'ts" section.

Growing her Hair to Long Lengths

Handle her hair very gently- use your fingers to separate the tangled ends of her hair.

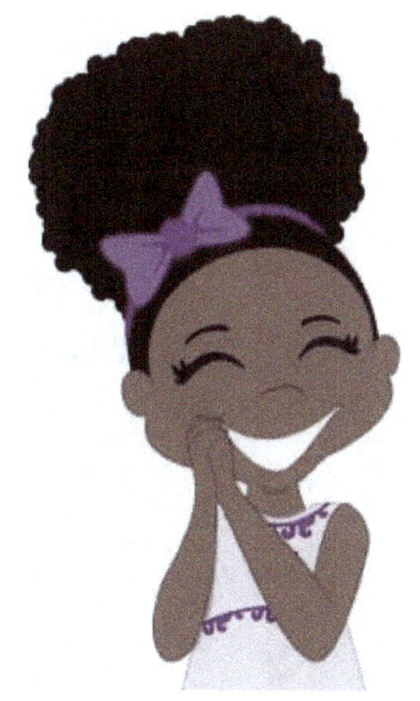

Review the steps from chapter 11 "Step By Step Guide on How to Wash African Textured Hair". Shampoo and condition her hair in twisted sections, *without* opening the twisted sections. No deep conditioning or scalp massages.

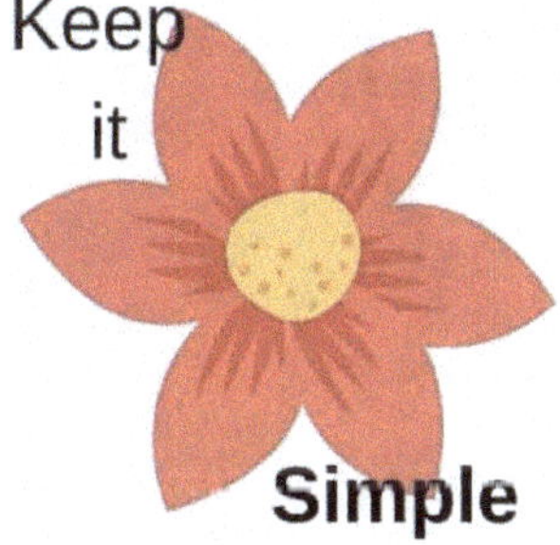

1) Do not use blow dryers or any heat on her hair.

2) For fine hair, use black crochet yarn to put medium twists in her hair because it is lighter and softer than synthetic hair. For thick hair, use natural looking synthetic hair or crochet yarn for her twists.

3) Keep her ends covered and protected in the twists.

4) Keep her twists style for 1-2 months.

5) Use the "Braid or twists with Extensions" monthly regimen to care for her hair while in the twists, but only wash and condition every two weeks.

6) Cover her hair at night (a stocking or pantyhose wrapped around her head may be more comfortable and secure).

7) Keep in mind that chlorine and salt water are very drying to her hair and can lead to breakage. If she has a school swimming program, do a "co-wash" that day when she gets home.

Most importantly: Tell her that her hair is beautiful....

CHAPTER 16

100% Natural Homemade
Hair Recipes

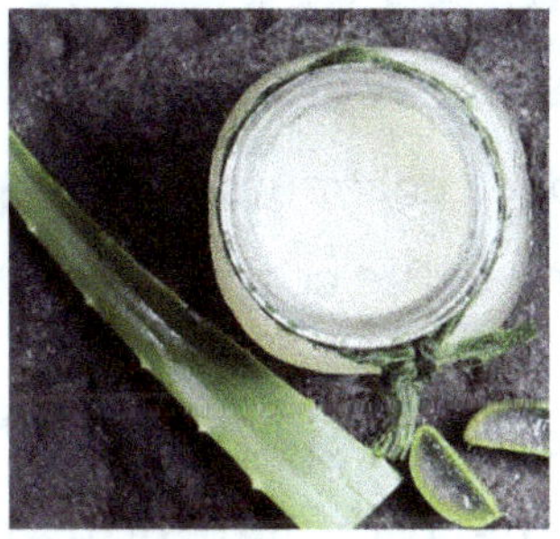

HOW TO MAKE ALOE VERA GEL AT HOME

a) Get one large aloe leaf (about the length of your forearm. Use 3 leaves if they are small.

b) Cut the bottom part (wider part of the leaf).

c) Lean the leaf to stand upright to allow to drain the green liquid from the part that has been cut.

d) Peel the leaf by cutting off the prickly edges, then slice off one of the flat green side of the leaf.

e) Lay the leaf down unto the uncut flat part of the leaf, then scrap off the white gel inside of the leaf and place into a bowl.

f) Use a fork or blender to mix the gel into a slimy liquid.

e) Pour gel into a glass bowl and refridgerate

◆ ◆ ◆

HOW TO MAKE COCONUT OIL AT HOME

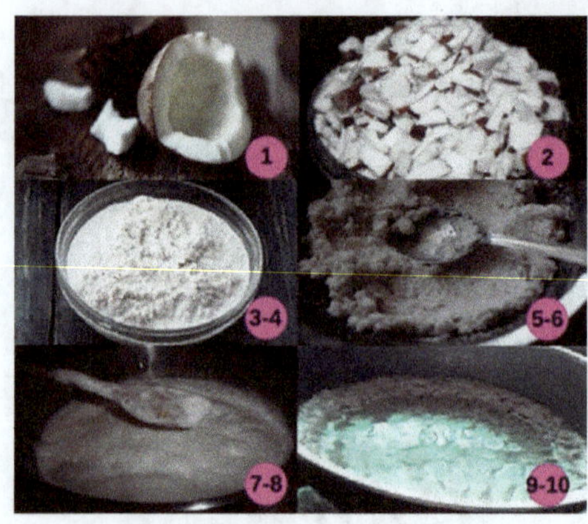

1) Get five fully developed coconuts.

2) Crack the shell, remove the coconut flesh, and cut into smaller pieces.

3) Blend or grind the coconut pieces.

4) Add warm water to the coconut to form a milky cake-like batter.

5) Using your hands, mix and squeeze the coconut to extract the coconut milk.

6) Use a cheese cloth or strainer to press and squeeze the liquid from the coconut pieces.

7) Cover the milky liquid in a container, at room temperature, for 24 hours or overnight. It will ferment. The next day, you will see a foam on the surface (this is the fermented part).

8) Carefully scrape the fermented part into a clean pot or pan.

9) Cook under very low heat and stir continuously. The fermented part will start separating and you will begin to see the coconut oil.

10) Store your coconut oil in a glass container. Cover tightly.

DEEP CONDITIONERS

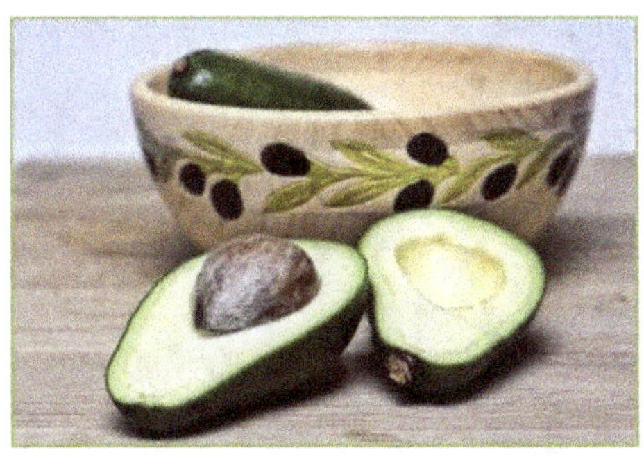

Directions for Use :

a) Mix all ingredients well before applying to your hair.

b) Apply to your hair, then cover with a plastic cap.

c) Use low heat under a hooded dryer. If you don't have one, use a small, warm, heated towel to wrap your head.

d) Leave treatment on your hair for 20-30 minutes.

c) Rinse hair, wait till your hair is almost dry, then apply your leave-in conditioner.

Moisturizing and Protein Deep Conditioner in One

2 eggs

1 medium avocado

1 1/2 teaspoons of olive oil, coconut oil, or castor oil

Aloe Vera & Honey Hair Mask (for Shiny Hair)

2-3 tablespoons of fresh aloe vera gel

2 tablespoons of yogurt

1 tablespoon of honey

1 tablespoon of castor, olive, or coconut oil

Banana Hair Mask (Softness and Shine)

(Blend immediately before use)

2 over-ripe bananas

3 tablespoons of honey

5 tablespoons of yogurt

◆ ◆ ◆

SCALP MASSAGE TREATMENTS

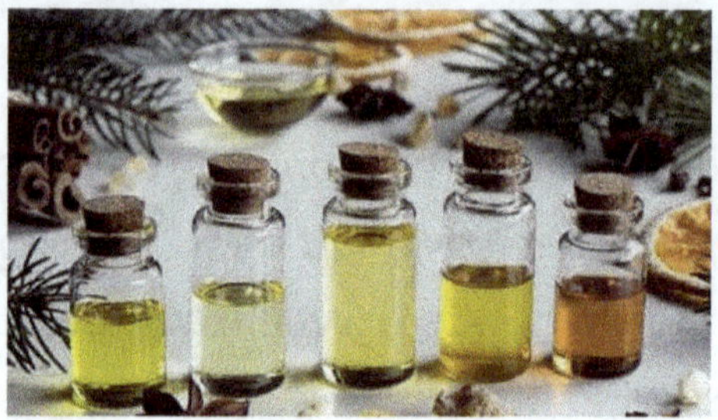

Directions for Use:

a) Massage in scalp for 10 minutes.

b) Wait 2 hours before your wash routine.

Onion Menthol Juice (to stimulate hair growth)

1 large onion (crushed, blended, and sieved)

3 drops of peppermint essential oil

Rosemary Infused Oil

1 cup of fresh rosemary

2 cups of liquid vegetable oil

Cook fresh rosemary in oil on very low heat, or 2-4 hours in a slow cooker on low. Let cool, then store away in glass container.

Carrot Juice & Black Cumin Seeds (Hair Thickness)

1/2 cup carrot juice

1 tablespoon black cumin powder

Guava Tea (Hair loss and Shedding)

2 cups of guava leaves

1 liter or 1 quart of water

**Boil leaves for 20 mins. Let cool.

◆ ◆ ◆

OIL TREATMENT

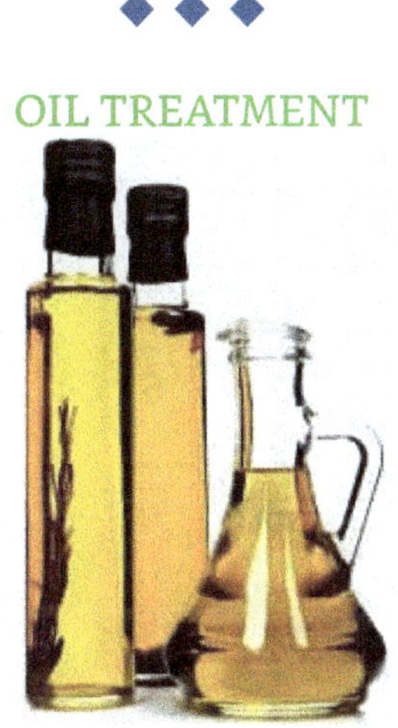

Hot Oil Treatment (for Soft Hair)

2 tablespoons coconut or castor oil

1 tablespoon jojoba oil or olive oil

3-5 drops of essential oil of your choice

1 small container to place your treatment

1 medium sized container (with a little bit of hot water) or use a pan of the stove top.

Directions for use:

a) Place the small container into the medium sized container of hot water, to safely heat the oils.

b) Keep checking until the oil gets warm, but not too hot or it will burn you.

c) Remove the warm oil, and apply throughout your hair and scalp.

d) Immediately cover your hair with a plastic cap, then apply a scarf or knitted hat over the plastic cap.

e) Remove after 30 minutes and rinse your hair in warm water, wait till your hair is almost dry, then apply your leave in conditioner.

RICE WATER TREATMENT

Rice Water (Softness and Shine)

3 cups of warm water (distilled)

1 cup of rice

Directions for Use:

a) Add rice to room temperature water.

b) Mix rice well, then cover in a pot, leave to ferment for 24 hours.

c) Use after shampoo/conditioning treatment. Apply to hair, cover with plastic cap for 30 minutes to one hour. Rinse and follow with your leave-in conditioner.

LEAVE-IN CONDITIONERS

Simple Leave-In Conditioner (Option 1)

1 cup of rose water

1/4 cup glycerin

Luxurious Leave-In Conditioner (Option 2)

2 tablespoons of above leave-in recipe

2 tablespoons of aloe vera juice

2 teaspoons of castor oil

2 teaspoons of coconut oil, olive oil, or avocado oil

Please check your hair type (Ch 6: Porosity and Thickness) to ensure that the recipes will be effective on your hair.

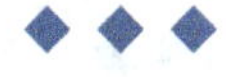

HENNA TREATMENT

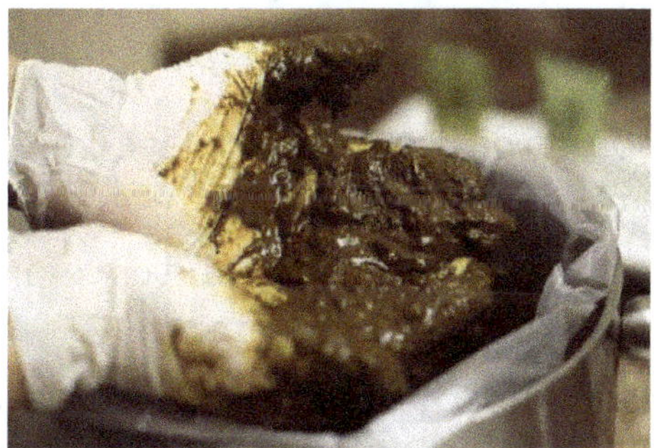

What is Henna?

Henna is produced from the leaves of the "henna plant". Once the leaves are obtained, they are crushed into a fine powder. The powder is then sifted and mixed with a variety of ingredients, such as essential oils.

How often should I use it?

Henna treatments are most effective when done in between long-term protective styling like braids or weaves. Every 6-8 weeks. If you choose to use henna, be sure that it is the pure henna and not the fake brands.

What benefits will henna have on my hair?

Natural henna allows the hair to be stronger and acts like a protein conditioner. The leaves also contain a red dye called "Lawsone", which essentially leaves a red tint on the hair (and anything else it touches).

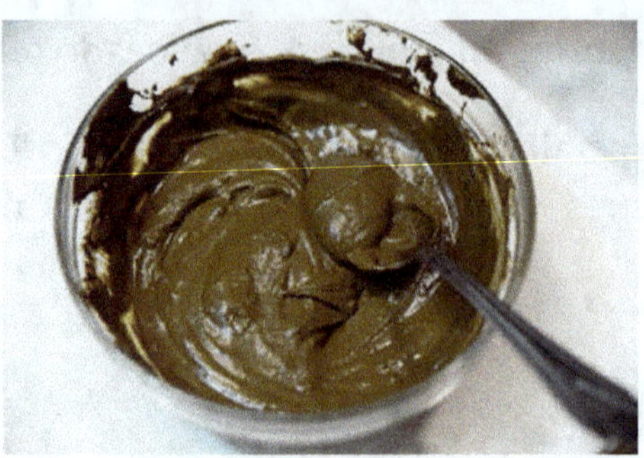

Directions for Use:

a) Mix a tablespoon of oil (coconut or olive), henna package and yogurt.

b) Form a consistency like cake batter and cover in a container the night before use. Keep at room temperature.

c) Shampoo your hair first then lightly dry with a towel so that it is not dripping wet.

d) Apply the mixture as you would a relaxer.

e) Leave on for one hour.

f) After rinsing, lightly towel dry and deep condition AGAIN for 30 mins using a MOISTURIZING TREATMENT. (This step is extremely important to reducing breakage after Henna treatment.)

e) Rinse and follow with your leave-in conditioner and oils.

ALLERGY WARNING: Product examples may contain ingredients that you may allergic to. Please do a small patch test before committing to using any product examples in this guide.

Rub the ingredient into the inner part of your arm, recheck the area after a few hours. If you notice any bumps or rashes, then this means you are allergic to this product and should not use it.

CAUTION: Henna is permanent. Adding commercial hair dye to hair that has had henna application could result in hair loss. Or make hair difficult to color with hair dye.

TIPS:

*Low porosity hair (chapter 6) should avoid henna.

*The oils you use will depend on your hair porosity (chapter 6).

*Milk is more moisturizing than lemon when used in henna.

A Final Thought

As women, part of our beauty, is our hair. In reality, it is a very small part of what it means to be beautiful. Our personalities, confidence, smile and body language say more about our beauty, than our hair. Even more important than all of these, is how we treat other people. Humility, kindness, honesty and grace, serves us well.

As you work towards your hair goals, know that it is only hair. Afro textured hair is a fun and unique feature for us. There is no right or wrong way to wear your hair. If you like it short, keep it short. If you think you would look good with a huge afro, then go ahead. If you want to use a texturizer, a relaxer, cut it off, then start over - go ahead. After all, your hair *will* grow back.

In the mean time, if you are trying to grow it long, then let it grow, and take good care of it.

Acknowledgements

First, I thank God for guiding me in the development and execution of *Grow Hair.* I want to express my appreciation to my editor, Jean Suren, for her great interest in, and enthusiasm for, this book and for bringing it into the world.

I also acknowledge all my friends and family for their support in America, Dominica, UK, Kenya, and around the world, too numerous to mention here, but who provide me with continual inspiration and encouragement.

As always, I would not have been able to complete this book without the unwavering support of my children – Xavier, Gabby, and Eli. They are my future.

Grow Hair is a guide for women of African textured hair to invest in and love their God given hair. To that extent, it would be remiss of me not to acknowledge all the women who without recognition work toward and respect the beauty that is our natural hair.

Thank You So Much!

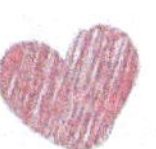 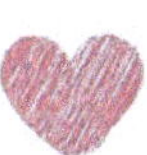 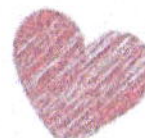

Select Bibliography

Etemesi, Beatrice Amunga. "Impact of hair relaxers in women in Nakuru, Kenya." International journal of dermatology 46.s1 (2007): 23-25.

Gavazzoni Dias, Maria Fernanda Reis. "Hair Cosmetics: An Overview." International Journal of Trichology 7.1 (2015): 2–15. PMC. Web. 29 Aug. 2017.

Khumalo, N. P., et al. "What is normal black African hair? A light and scanning electron-microscopic study." Journal of the American Academy of Dermatology 43.5 (2000): 814-820.

Loussouarn, G. "African hair growth parameters." British Journal of Dermatology 145.2 (2001): 294-297.

Olsen, Elise A., et al. "Central hair loss in African American women: incidence and potential risk factors." Journal of the American Academy of Dermatology 64.2 (2011): 245-252.

Shapiro, Jerry. "Hair loss in women." New England Journal of Medicine 357.16 (2007): 1620-1630.

Sperling, Leonard C. "Hair density in African Americans." Archives of dermatology 135.6 (1999): 656-658.

T Chiu, Chin-Hsien, Shu-Hung Huang, and Hui-Min D Wang. "A review: Hair health, concerns of shampoo ingredients and scalp nourishing treatments." Current pharmaceutical biotechnology 16.12 (2015): 1045-1052.

Trüeb, Ralph M. "Pharmacologic Interventions in Aging Hair." Clinical Interventions in Aging 1.2 (2006): 121–129. Print.

Wise, Lauren A., et al. "Hair relaxer use and risk of uterine leiomyomata in African-American women." American journal of epidemiology 175.5 (2012): 432-440.

www.ingramcontent.com/pod-product-compliance
Lightning Source LLC
Chambersburg PA
CBHW050048260726
48658CB00005B/1836